U82

2.50

BEHIND THE BLUE DOOR
The History of The Royal College of Midwives
1881-1981

This book is to be returned on or before the last date stamped below.

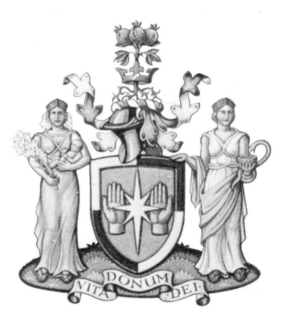

The coat of arms of the Royal College of Midwives

Facing page: The old 'Vita Donum Dei' badge devised for the members of the Midwives' Institute in 1941

BEHIND THE BLUE DOOR

The History of the Royal College of Midwives

1881-1981

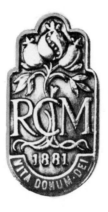

Betty Cowell and David Wainwright

Baillière Tindall · London

Published with the support of Colgate Palmolive Ltd
makers of Curity Snugglers

A BAILLIÈRE TINDALL book published by
Cassell Ltd. £2.50
35 Red Lion Square, London WC1R 4SG
and at Sydney, Auckland, Toronto, Johannesburg
an affiliate of Macmillan Publishing Co., Inc.,
New York

Text and illustrations © The Royal College of Midwives 1981

First published 1981

ISBN 0 7020 0881 8

Typeset by Inforum Ltd.
Printed and bound by Richard Clay (The Chaucer Press) Ltd,
Bungay, Suffolk.

Contents

Acknowledgements

The authors wish to record their thanks to the present and past members of the Royal College of Midwives who have generously given their time and interest to contribute to the making of this book.

B.C. and D.W., London, January 1981

CLARENCE HOUSE
S.W. 1

As Patron, I am delighted to have this opportunity of sending my greetings and congratulations on the occasion of the centenary of the Royal College of Midwives.

During the past one hundred years many new skills have been developed and new techniques have been acquired. Much has changed but the high professional standards of the College have always been most worthily maintained.

This landmark in the history of the College is, however, also a time for looking forward. I am confident that the College will continue to play its very important rôle in caring for mothers and babies and in giving advice and guidance to midwives.

I send to you all my warmest good wishes for the years ahead.

ELIZABETH R
Queen Mother

Foreword

The Royal College of Midwives is indebted to all those who have made it possible for every member of the College to receive this book as a gift during the centenary year. My thanks go to Colgate Palmolive – makers of Curity Snugglers – for their generous sponsorship of the book, to Betty Cowell and David Wainwright for their skill in writing it, and to Bounty Services Limited for their vision in seeking sponsorship for it and distributing it.

It now remains for me to invite all those who read the book to enjoy the unfolding of a story which combines the delights of the familiar with the excitement of the unfamiliar or forgotten.

DOROTHY M. WEBSTER, SRN SCM MTD.
President of the Royal College of Midwives

February 1981

ONE

The Fight for Legislation

On an autumn day in 1876 an elegantly-dressed woman walked through the slums of Seven Dials, then one of the worst areas of housing in central London, lying between Shaftesbury Avenue and Trafalgar Square. She was Louisa Hubbard, proprietor and editor of a woman's journal called *Work and Leisure*. She was being guided by a younger woman, less fashionably dressed but well-educated and articulate. This was Zepherina Veitch, who was working as a midwife among the poor, from her base at the British Lying-in Hospital nearby in Endell Street.

In the previous year, Miss Hubbard had published a series of articles, written with the cooperation of Florence Nightingale, on 'Nursing as a Profession for Educated Women'. Miss Veitch had read them, realised that this was an excellent platform on which to mount her own personal campaign to improve the standards of midwifery, and written an article which she sent to *Work and Leisure*. Miss Hubbard was impressed by it (and published it in December 1876); but being the woman she was, she took steps to meet the author and see her work at first hand.

Miss Veitch impressed her profoundly, as she did all who met her. The elder daughter of a clergyman, she had trained as a nurse under the All Saints' Sisters at University College Hospital. She then in 1868 took charge of the surgical wards at King's College Hospital, and a year later was appointed Superintendent of Nurses at St George's Hospital.

In the following year, the Franco-Prussian War having broken out, she nursed with the All Saints' Sisters at Sedan. On her return in 1871 she became Sister-in-charge at Charing Cross Hospital; but she became increasingly concerned with the situation then prevailing in midwifery, particularly among the poor. No impoverished woman could afford the guinea fee required then by the doctors, and so she was thrown back for aid on the army of local midwives, many of whom practised a sort of folk-magic, their 'skill', when it existed, being handed down often from mother to daughter. The worst of them were caricatured by Charles Dickens in Sairey Gamp, and he did not over-exaggerate.

There was no control over these midwives; and while some were effective practitioners, others caused frightful mortality when faced with some abnormality and would sometimes abandon their patients to agony and death. There can be no doubt that in many cases, particularly in the crowded dwellings of urban slums, these women directly spread disease and infection. Zepherina Veitch saw that the answer to this social evil lay in the proper training of midwives, and then their control by legislation.

It was skill and knowledge that Miss Veitch wanted to spread. Despite her own nursing experience, she herself undertook a course of training in midwifery at the British Lying-in Hospital, Endell Street, and, qualifying in January 1873, obtained the diploma of the London Obstetrical Society (she was only the tenth person to hold it). Then she began her work in the slums. It is recorded that on her first visit to an out-patient, she found that 'the mother was in a condition of the direst poverty, and that there was nothing in the house larger than an Australian meat tin in which the baby could have its first wash. But Miss Veitch, who had lived in Palestine, and had learned how to rough it in the deserts of the Holy Land, speedily solved the difficulty by making a bath in her own lap out of the big waterproof apron she wore.'

She was convinced of the need to support compassion with trained skill and in approaching Miss Hubbard she took the first step towards achieving that aim. Louisa Maria Hubbard was a woman of her time, and in her way one of the most extraordinary innovators and campaigners of that day. If her work today seems anachronistic, it is largely because she herself set in train the social transformation that has made it so. It must be remembered that when she was young, in the 1840s, the idea of middle-class daughters being formally educated or trained in any skill was considered inappropriate, and certainly not 'ladylike'. Daughters might learn 'household management' and the domestic skills that would fit them for marriage. They might be taught undemanding leisure pursuits such as a little light needlework, watercolour painting, or playing the piano in an amateur way. Then they would marry and put their abilities to social use within the family. The attitude persisted, for when late in 1876 Zepherina Veitch married the distinguished surgeon Professor Henry Smith she was obliged to give up her own career, though as 'Mrs Henry Smith' she entered into the annals of midwifery as the foremost authority of the time.

Not all Victorian daughters married. Those who did not could find themselves in dire straits unless they were backed by substantial inheritances, being without the training to earn their own living. Hence there grew up an army of 'governesses', many of them impoverished gentlewomen patronised by the families they served. There were plenty of single ladies in Victorian England – the 'sisters and cousins and aunts' of W.S Gilbert's verse.

Louisa Hubbard could not see why the energies and talents of this battalion of single women should not be put to good use; good for them, and good for society. She was concerned for them, because she was one of them herself. Born in St Petersburg in 1836 of a wealthy British family trading in Russia, she grew up there before returning to her father's Sussex estate.

There was therefore no financial or social pressure on Louisa Hubbard to do more than lead the conventional life of one sustained by extreme wealth. This from the first she declined to do. She was drawn into good works in her late twenties. A friend at some fashionable London drawing-room invited

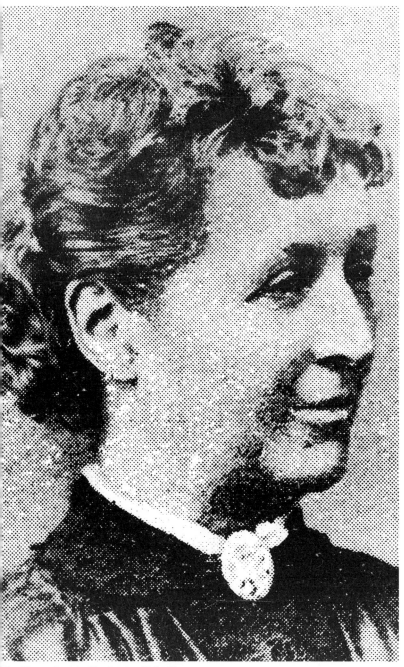

Mrs Henry Smith (Zepherina Veitch)

her to go and visit the Deaconesses in Burton Crescent. The Primitive Order of Deaconesses had been founded three years earlier, in 1861, by Miss Catherine Ferard, who had been trained at Kaiserwerth in Germany (Florence Nightingale had also been influenced by that movement, though she was unimpressed by their nursing standards). The purpose was to provide a body of women trained in nursing, teaching, and aiding the poor, to assist the clergy of the Church of England in the congested urban parishes. Louisa Hubbard was impressed by the movement, and determined to help it first by organising a series of fund-raising 'assistance meetings' among her wealthy friends, and secondly by writing to the Press. She found she could write effectively.

She took up the cause, following the Elementary Education Act of 1870 of training 'ladies' as school teachers, and helped to found a training college for them (Otter College, Chichester). The flood of applications for places confirmed her view that the many thousands of unmarried women in the country were a largely untapped source of social wealth for the community. In 1875 she published a *Handbook for Women's Work*, which she was to edit annually for eighteen years; and in that year too she founded a journal which she called *Woman's Gazette* (the title was later changed to *Work and Leisure*).

Louisa Hubbard early realised what the suffragettes and trade unionists of the next generation were to work on so powerfully, an awareness that people with a common interest could advance their cause by associating together in societies, and by communicating with each other through the printed word. She founded a Working Ladies' Guild, a Teachers' Guild, a Society for Housing Working Gentlewomen, and a Women's Friendly Society; and she gave them all a voice in her journal.

It was inevitable that early in her public career Louisa Hubbard should meet Florence Nightingale, and be impressed by her powerful campaign for the improvement of nursing standards. Her work was, by chance, done at a time of notable advances in medical knowledge (most notably the use of anaesthesia at childbirth by Sir James Simpson, the work of Lister on antiseptics, and of Pasteur). A further trend – though not one of which Miss Nightingale approved – was the increasing demand for the emancipation of women.

Some years previously the Medical Act of 1858 had been passed; this was to come into effect in 1886, and under it registration as a medical practitioner was dependent on a qualification in midwifery as well as medicine and surgery. It was only natural that this qualification was jealously guarded by men, who strongly opposed any attempt by women to qualify equally with them in the practice of medicine, and it was not until 1876 that the General Medical Council agreed to accept women for registration.

It was in this year, and this climate, that Louisa Hubbard published Zepherina Veitch's article on the improvement of midwifery standards. Though the article provoked considerable discussion, it was to be four years before positive action followed. In May 1880 Louisa Hubbard published in *Work and Leisure* a list of those sixteen women who had to that date gained medical qualification and earned their place on the British Medical Register. The Matron of a Sheffield hospital (Mrs E. Hornby Evans of the Jessop Hospital) wrote to suggest that it would be useful if a similar list of professionally qualified midwives could be published, since this would probably demonstrate how few there were, and could be the means of encouraging midwives to take training. Typically, Louisa Hubbard introduced Mrs Evans to Mrs Henry Smith. They also discussed the problem with Dr James Aveling and with the London Obstetrical Society (which had instituted its diploma by examination eight years earlier). The list was published in *Work and Leisure* for November 1880; it contained sixty-three names.

Dr James Aveling was a founding member of the London Obstetrical Society, founder of the *Obstetrical Journal*, and a founder of the Chelsea Hospital for Women, of which he was at this time resident physician. In 1872 he had published a standard work on midwifery, and was a powerful advocate of training. A pupil of Sir James Simpson the pioneer of anaesthesia, he began practice in Sheffield, it is said, because the wife of the vicar of the parish wanted a doctor there trained to administer chloroform during childbirth. That was a controversial matter in 1852, though the opposition was stifled when in the following year Queen Victoria accepted chloroform at the birth of her eighth child.

Dr Aveling wanted midwives to be better trained, though even he did not believe that women should aspire to medical qualifications. He supported the nomination of Elizabeth Garrett Anderson for admission to the London Obstetrical Society, but said that he did not plead the cause of women as obstetricians, 'because I think, if there is one operation for which they are less fitted than another, it is that of attending the emergencies of obstetric practice'. Women might take the examinations and qualify for the Society's certificate, but they could not become members. In 1881, Dr Aveling was chairman of the examining board, and thus an obvious authority for Louisa Hubbard to consult.

Typically, Miss Hubbard was not content to be simply a catalyst; she must organise a practical society. While the list of midwives was being compiled, a meeting was held at the offices of *Work and Leisure* at 42 Somerset Street in the autumn of 1881. It was attended by Mrs Smith, Mrs Evans (the Sheffield matron), Miss King (secretary of the Society for Promoting the Employment of Women), Miss Hubbard and others. It was agreed that a society was needed; thus, in October 1881, Miss Hubbard published an announcement of the imminent formation of a society to be called the 'Matron's Aid, or Trained Midwives' Registration Society'.

The prospectus was briskly factual:

'Out of 1,250,000 births which take place in Great Britain annually it is calculated that only about 3 in 10 are at present attended by medical men. This was stated in 1869 by a Committee appointed by the Council of the Obstetrical Society to investigate the causes of infant mortality, and another equally good authority reduces the number to 1 in 10. From 7 to 9 births in 10, or over 1,000,000 annually, are therefore attended by women only. These women are under no control or regulation whatever in England . . . In countries where midwives only are employed the proportion to the population is 1 for 2000. Allowing for the present rate of attendance in lying-in cases by medical men in this country it is calculated that about 10,000 midwives are required. To meet this demand only 80 women at present hold a certificate of any value.

'In addition, therefore, to the argument that an increase in the number of trained and licensed midwives is absolutely needed, a larger adoption of this calling would afford maintenance to the numbers of women who need to earn a livelihood, from £80 (which is easily earned in fees in towns, even among the poorer class), to several hundreds a year in the Colonies, or where midwives practice among the wealthy, being obtainable.'

The prospectus was sent to Florence Nightingale, who replied on 1 September 1881:

'I cannot express the very great interest which I take in the subject upon which you have been so good as to write to me, nor the joy with which I hail any step towards an attempt to deal with it, or even to direct attention to it. If I refer to a poor little book I once published, *Notes on Lying-in Institution* which you may possibly have read, it is only to save your trouble and mine, and to try, on so vast a subject, not to write a book in a letter. The main object of the *'Notes'* was (after dealing with the sanitary question) to point out the utter absence of any means of training in any existing institutions in Great Britain. Since the *'Notes'* were written, next to nothing has been done to remedy this defect . . . The prospectus appears to contain much that is most excellent . . . I wish you success from the bottom of my heart if, as I cannot doubt, your wisdom and energy work out a scheme by which to supply the *deadly* want of training among women practising midwifery in England. (It is a farce and a mockery to call them midwives or even midwifery nurses, and no certificate now given makes them so). France Germany and even Russia would consider it *woman*- slaughter to 'practise' as we do . . . It is true that in these countries everything is done by Government; with us by private enterprise. But we are not accustomed in England to hold private enterprise as lagging behind Government in efficiency.'

Much encouraged by this eminent support, a meeting was held on 10 December 1881 and the 'Matron's Aid Society, or Trained Midwives Registration Society' was in being. Miss Hubbard, who had been organising secretary, handed over that role to Mrs Bedingfield, a trained midwife. Other supporters on that occasion were Miss Jane Wilson and Miss Free man, the Matron of the British Lying-in Hospital.

It must be admitted that no great social change followed. The ten or a dozen of the twenty-six members of the Society, those working in London would meet from time to time at Miss Hubbard's house or that of Mrs

Henry Smith. The objects of the Society were to promote a thorough training of women as midwives, to keep a register, and to offer to those who were thoroughly trained and certificated the advantage of an association for mutual support and benefit.

For the first four years, the last seems to have been the most practical achievement of the Society. In part this was no doubt because of the constraints on the two chief founders: Miss Hubbard was not a qualified midwife (and indeed somewhat abashed by the very word, which was not customarily spoken in her social world), and Mrs Henry Smith, who was qualified, felt constrained not to embarrass her husband whose professional career could have been irreparably damaged by public controversy or any suspicion of 'advertising', a heinous offence among Victorian doctors.

Then in the spring of 1886 Miss Freeman, Matron of the British Lying-in Hospital, found the person who was to put the Society firmly and vigorously on the right road. She was a newly-qualified young midwife, Rosalind Paget.

In later years Dame Rosalind recalled:

'After taking my L.O.S. (London Obstetrical Society certificate) . . . I was walked off to one of their meetings by my Matron, Miss Freeman. It was at Mrs Smith's house (in Wimpole Street). There were about ten persons present, and it was very dull. At the end the Secretary said would I join. I said: "No, I think not, but if you have a Midwives' Club and lectures and a library, I will." Next day I was asked to help them organise one; this was the beginning of the Midwives' Institute as it now is. Mrs Henry Smith was our inspiration, Miss Wilson provided the brains, and I was the legs that did the running about for them.'

Rosalind Paget was a dedicated nurse. She had grown up in Liverpool, at the house of her uncle William Rathbone, who had virtually introduced the idea and practice of district nursing in that congested and feverish city. 'She was endowed,' writes Mary Stocks, 'with Rathbone energy, intelligence and restless social conscience'. Against the wishes of her family, she worked as a nurse in Liverpool and Manchester.

Then she came to London and was trained at the London Hospital, and then gained the certificate of the London Obstetrical Society after working at the Lying-in Hospital. No doubt her driving energy was what appealed to Matron Freeman; but her social contacts cannot have been unhelpful, when allied to such unquestioned professional skill.

The first change was to put the lectures on to a professional footing. No longer were they held in drawing-rooms; a room was booked on Friday evenings at 22 Berners Street. It was there, in April 1886, that Dr Hugh Fenton lectured to an audience of seventy on 'puerperal sepsis'. There were still only fifteen certificated members, but evidently Miss Paget had put the word round to good effect. In June, a room was taken as an office at 15 Buckingham Street, the headquarters of the Charity Organisation Society, and a series of lectures was planned for certificated midwives and trained nurses. The lectures were given by doctors and other staff from the London Hospital (where Rosalind Paget had trained).

Unfortunately there was growing antagonism to the Institute from the medical profession. It was averred that the medical lectures given there, and then published in *Nursing Notes*, were a breach of regulations of the Royal Colleges and were akin to advertising. The London Hospital doctors had hastily to withdraw, and that summer's lectures were given by friends of the Institute willing to take the risk of professional ostracism.

With the move to Buckingham Street the name of the society was changed to the 'Midwives' Institute and Trained Nurses' Club', thus acknowledging its true purpose. Louisa Hubbard was less closely linked with it, in part because she travelled abroad for her health (she suffered a stroke while in the Austrian Tyrol in 1889, and remained there until her death in 1906). She referred to her 'immature efforts' in helping to found the Institute; but she deserves to be more generously remembered for seeing the need for such a body, and helping to establish it.

Having arranged the medical lectures on a more formal basis, Rosalind Paget set about the business of communication among the midwives around the country. On 1 June 1887 there was published the first issue of *Nursing Notes*, a four-page supplement to the journal *Woman*. That first issue opened with Miss Paget's clear vision of the need for it:

'Ever since Miss Nightingale's noble work in the Crimea, trained nursing has been an acknowledged necessity. The institution which has for thirty years been a fitting memorial of her labours, is now only one among many similar ones which annually add to the numbers of trained, intelligent, often highly-educated women, who devote their lives to nursing the sick, either as hospital sisters and nurses, as parish or district nurses in workhouse infirmaries among the poor, or in the private houses of the rich.

'The class of certificated midwives is also on the increase, and will in time supersede the untrained woman in that branch of work. All these women when they have finished their various training in the hospitals are, perhaps, for the first time fully aware how much still remains to learn. Indeed, no nurse can ever feel anything but a learner all her life. As the resources of medical science will never cease, so nursing is a work where there are constantly some new devices for the alleviation of suffering. The fullest term of training only fits the nurse really to know how vast is the field open to her. It is the alphabet and grammar of her new language; its literature is still before her. While she is still an inmate of the Hospital, the opportunities she enjoys of benefiting by the instructions and lectures of physicians, and the daily example and teaching of the experienced sister of her ward, would render these papers almost superfluous, especially as many of the hospitals provide medical papers and libraries of valuable books for the use of the nurses.

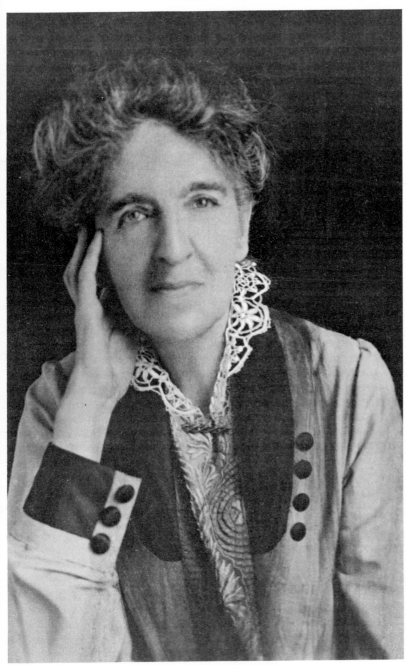

Dame Roslind Paget (1855–1948), a leader of the Midwives' Institute

But the case is different when the nurse is sent to private or district nursing, or as a midwife begins to practise. In the country 24, and sometimes 48 hours may elapse between the doctor's visits, even in dangerous cases, and still longer intervals in chronic cases, which depend mainly on nursing . . . 'It is one of the serious drawbacks to the nursing profession that many of its most interesting details, to those who are trained to understand them, are either uninteresting or unpleasant to the outside world, and the nurse must always on leaving the hospital sadly miss the pleasant intercourse she has hitherto enjoyed with the sisters and her fellow probationers, and it is then we hope she will turn to these pages to keep up with the nursing world and for a while to associate in spirit with those who are sharing her work. If this is true of the trained nurse, it is far more so of the certified midwife whose work is almost always alone, and who does not return, as the private nurse sometimes does, to the intercourse of the Home or Hospital. We hope every month to present to those readers an account of the proceedings of the Midwives' Institute and Trained Nurses' Club with reports of the very interesting lectures delivered from time to time by eminent doctors interested in this branch of the profession.'

That summer, it was announced at the General Meeting of the Institute that the membership had risen from 26 to 170. Miss Paget was well aware that the membership was largely to be found in London, and that if the Institute was to achieve its aims, it must widen its appeal throughout the country in the growing towns and in the impoverished rural areas hard hit by the agricultural depression.

Nursing Notes was to be the means of speaking to that dispersed audience. It did not have an easy beginning because after it had only been in existence for a few months as a supplement to *Woman*, that journal merged with another, and it became necessary to make other arrangements. In January 1888 it was launched on its independent course by an editor and proprietor, Emma Brierly, who for thirty-five years made it her life's work. She was the daughter of Sir Oswald Brierly, marine painter to Queen Victoria; throughout the years when the Midwives' Institute was fighting for formal recognition, she spent her time and her income on the support of its cause.

When *Nursing Notes* became independent it chose to be produced by the Women's Printing Society Limited, since it was thought that 'a paper written entirely for one branch of women's work ought if possible to support another branch of women's work'. Emma Brierly was quietly determined; a colleague remembered that on occasions when she was discussing with Miss Paget 'some of the absorbing happenings of the moment', time and again 'Miss Brierly would bring us back to editorial duties with the dry little remark, "And now, dear ladies, may we *once* more come back to business?" '.

Miss Brierly not only edited the journal, she acted as advertising manager too. It was the first journal of its kind and though it never made a profit, an early member of the staff recalled:

'When *Nursing Notes* was started there were *no* nursing papers, and the word midwife was taboo, but *Nursing Notes*, though chiefly supported by trained nurses from its first number gave the Midwives' Institute a space for its reports, had its office under the same roof, and though keeping the paper independent and under a quite separate Editorial Committee, began that close friendship with the Midwives' Institute which has lasted without a rift for nearly forty years.'

Nursing Notes showed a loss on its first year of some £8 which 'owing to a small reserve fund in charge of the treasurer we were able to meet'. The treasurer was Rosalind Paget and no doubt the small reserve fund was her own pocket.

It was clearly necessary to make sure that the Institute was founded in the most formal way. In 1889 it was incorporated under the Companies' Act. With incorporation, the purposes of the Institute became more strongly defined:

1. To raise the efficiency and improve the status of Midwives, and to petition Parliament for their recognition.
2. To establish a registry for Members and a centre of information for the public.
3. To provide a good Medical Lending Library and Club-room for friendly meetings.
4. To arrange courses of Medical Lectures and to afford opportunities for discussion on subjects connected with the profession.

The need to petition Parliament had become paramount. Two Bills for the registration of midwives had been drafted some years earlier by the London Obstetrical Society, and though discussed favourably by the British Medical Association had not achieved sufficient support to merit parliamentary consideration. The men had failed to act. Now their sisters and cousins and aunts (and wives) would try.

A 'drawing-room' meeting was held at the house of Mrs. Rathbone, in Princes Gardens, in May 1889. Lady Rosebery and the Countess of Aberdeen sent apologies for absence, but Lady Aberdare, Lady FitzWygram, Lady Knutsford and Lady Gibbs were present, with a host of untitled society ladies (among them, Mrs Oscar Wilde). Louisa Hubbard, on her last appearance for this cause, urged legislation, and it was agreed to pursue this. A vote of thanks was proposed by Dr. Annie McCall – not a member of the Institute, since she had qualified as a doctor (in Dublin, Switzerland and Vienna); but she specialised in midwifery, and that January had opened the Clapham Maternity Hospital and School of Midwifery.

Though *Nursing Notes* was edited from the premises of the Midwives' Institute, it gave news of a variety of activities, among them those of the Workhouse Infirmary Association (the particular interest of Jane Wilson), the Society of Trained Masseuses, the Royal National Pension Fund for Nurses, and others. The journal gave much space to matters concerning midwives (so much, in fact, that some nurses complained about this obsession); but it also described the development of the Queen's Institute nursing scheme. This had grown from the fund collected by the women of Britain to mark the Jubilee of Queen Victoria, who in 1887 celebrated fifty years on the throne.

When the Committee looked for someone who could breathe life into this new organisation, and knit together the multiplicity of local nursing schemes, one name came to the fore: Rosalind Paget. It was said of her (by the Lady Superintendent of the London Hospital) that she worked 'with equal success in charge of medical, surgical, accident and obstetric wards. She had attended operations of almost every description and her efficiency had been mentioned with special praise by different surgeons'. She was interested in teaching, and had been sympathetic in dealing with the sick poor.

Miss Paget was determined not to accept a salary, but since she did not want to be branded an amateur do-gooder, she agreed to be appointed Inspector General of the Queen's Institute at a salary of £100 a year, which she gave back to the Institute. Though she insisted that she would not do the job for more than a year or two, she typically spent the last months of 1889 as an ordinary probationer with the Metropolitan and National Nursing Association. When the Roll of Queen's Nurses was opened in January 1890, the first name was that of Rosalind Paget. She was to be Inspector until September 1891, but at the request of the Queen she became a member of the Institute's Council.

In August 1889 *Nursing Notes* reported that 'we cannot express the satisfaction we feel in being able at last to announce that among the Parliamentary Notices for next session, Mr. Henry Fell Pease will introduce a Bill for the Registration of Midwives'. It was to be a Private Member's Bill. Well-wishers had raised £1,000 towards the campaign. The prevalent optimism was supported by a resolution passed by the General Medical Council in December:

'This Council regards the absence of public provision for the education and supervision of midwives as productive of a large amount of grave suffering and fatal disease among the poorer classes, and urges upon the Government the importance of passing into law some measure for the education and registration of midwives.'

This was given additional strength by a letter of support signed by a dozen of the leading consultant obstetrical physicians at the London hospitals, including two past presidents of the London Obstetrical Society, one of them the distinguished Robert Barnes of St George's Hospital, founder of the Society. Three other signatories were to remain staunch supporters over the years – Graily Hewitt (University College Hospital), Francis Champneys (St George's) and Charles James Cullingworth (St Thomas's).

However, enthusiasm fell away as the Bill proceeded, until it came up for its second reading on 21 May 1890. It was opposed by a Dr Tanner (ironically, an Irish Member for Mid Cork, since the Bill did not apply to Ireland) who said that 'he had received representations from medical men stating that the passage of this Bill would deprive them of much legitimate practice which they at present enjoyed'.

That was the straightforward objection made by some country doctors – that the registered midwives at half-a-guinea would undercut the guinea-a-visit doctors. Other objections were more abstruse. Mr. J.T. Brunner said that the Bill required that every woman registered should be of good moral character:

'He objected to that most strongly (*loud laughter*), and thought that if women were to require such certificates men should be required to have the same.'

Charles Bradlaugh also opposed because 'they were striving to interfere too much in every department of life'. Dentists, opticians now had to register. Who next?

These objections were not flippant. These worries were shared by many who supported the principle of registration, since the controls laid down by the draft Bill were a complicated compromise. There was to be a London Midwives' Board consisting of the senior obstetricians of eleven London hospitals, with one representative each from the three medical corporations, the London Obstetrical Society, the University of London, and the Midwives' Institute. The General Medical Council would establish the rules for examination, registration and discipline. The London board would supervise provincial boards; but the governance of the scheme would be wholly in the hands of doctors, and entirely male.

The Bill was given a second reading on 7 July and referred to a Select Committee. In September it was blocked at the third reading owing to shortage of time, and withdrawn.

The doctors' view was expressed by a sub-committee of the British Medical Association:

'The standpoint from which we all started was that it had been universally agreed by the Medical Council, by the Parliamentary Bills Committee and by the Association in accepting the reports of that committee, that there was a great necessity for restricting and regulating the practice of midwives, and for providing that no persons should assume the title who were not properly educated. Then came the question of what was the best method of carrying it out. The first difficulty was as to the authorities for restricting and regulating midwives, and for creating a register. In that respect we were thoroughly dissatisfied with Mr Pease's bill . . .

The Government were also dissatisfied with the authorities proposed to be created. We also complained that the Bill did not prescribe limits for the practice of midwives, and did not provide the means for discipline in case of the infraction of any of the limits which the Bill might lay down.'

They agreed that the Bill should be recast at once. The General Medical Council was to have the authority to prescribe first of all what should be the general limits of practice of midwives; second, what should be the curriculum of education; third, how the examination should be conducted, where they should be conducted and what means should be taken to render the examinations uniform; the whole was to be subject to the Privy Council. The Government proposed that while the GMC should regulate, it was the duty of County Councils to provide places for examinations, to take charge of registration, and to provide funds. All persons in bona fide practice at the time of the Act were to be registered, but with a recommendation or certificate from a registered practitioner, and a testimony of good character.

The Government was now well aware of general concern over this subject. The word 'midwife' was no longer taboo, but on the contrary was appearing again and again on the Parliamentary agenda. The Bill was put down again for its second reading on 22 January 1891, but postponed to 5 March due to lack of time. On 27 February the Lord President of the Council (Lord Cranbrook) received a deputation of representatives of the BMA, the London Obstetrical Society and the British Gynaecological Society, but was dismissive: the Government could not support a bill that year. There was no time for the Bill on 5 March; it was put down three times for second reading in June, but never reached.

In 1890 the Midwives' Institute moved across Buckingham Street from No. 15 to No. 12. This part of London is replete with literary and political associations. At No. 15 (now the home of the Royal National Pension Fund for Nurses), Peter the Great of Russia is said to have lived, from its windows studying the movements of shipping. At No. 12, Sir Walter Scott is said to have written *The Talisman* (in what was to become the midwives' clubroom); Charles Dickens is said to have occupied part of the house, and it was here that Betsy Trotwood took the top room for David Copperfield when he entertained Mr. and Mrs. Micawber to supper. The move of the Midwives' Institute to No. 12 was severely practical. A small room was rented daily from 2 p.m., and a larger room for meetings on Friday evenings. From 1891 two rooms were taken full-time (one became the office, the other the members' room). In 1894 they added a lecture room and a little tea room, and later a small committee room or smoking room. The Institute was thus equipped both as a meeting place and a centre of information.

Meanwhile the Midwives' Institute was continuing the campaign for a training and registration. In October 1890 the Institute announced 'courses of lectures for the preparation of candidates for the Obstetrical examination are given weekly throughout the year. Members of the Institute can attend the classes at greatly reduced fees. No pupil prepared at the Midwives' Institute has as yet failed to pass the examination'. In July 1891 the Institute published a pamphlet listing those midwives who had passed the LOS examination from 1872 to 1891. It contained over 1,000 names. This demonstrated, of course, that the basis for a fully qualified midwifery profession already existed.

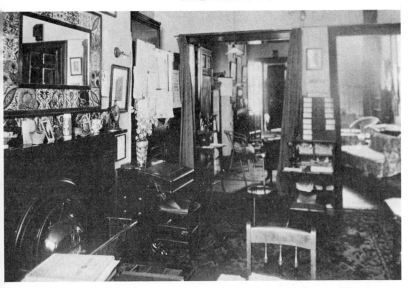

The first club-room of the Midwives' Institute at Buckingham Street. The tiles around the mirror, by William de Morgan, are still in the possession of the Royal College

The proposal for registration was now being vehemently opposed by two groups: a group of provincial general practitioners, the most articulate of whom was Dr Robert Rentoul of Liverpool, and the British Nurses' Association, founded in 1887 by Mrs Bedford Fenwick (a former Matron of St. Bartholomew's Hospital) to campaign for the registration of nurses. Mrs Fenwick, having failed to ally the Midwives' Institute to her cause, branded midwives as 'an anachronism' and a 'historical curiosity' in her journal the *Nursing Record*.

The bitter antagonism of the various sides in this dispute enabled successive Governments to claim that there could be no legislation while those most closely concerned, the doctors, nurses and midwives, were so implacably divided. In March 1892, however, a Select Committee of the House of Commons was appointed to look into the matter, and it met in May. Among those who gave evidence were Rosalind Paget and Mrs Henry Smith. Before the Select Committee could make its formal report, the Government resigned, and there was a General Election. In an interim report, the Committee said that the present position was unsatisfactory, called for legislation, reported the evidence, and sought leave to sit again in the new Parliament.

It sat again in the summer of 1893, and heard evidence from Dr Annie McCall, and Mrs Elinor Agnes Bedingfield – first secretary of the Midwives' Institute, a qualified midwife. When the Select Committee reported in August 1893, it was unequivocal:

'A large number of maternal and particularly infant deaths, as well as a serious amount of suffering and permanent injury to women and children, is caused from the inefficiency and want of skill of many of the women practising as midwives, without proper training and qualification. The Committee find that amongst the poor and working classes, both in the country and in the towns, the services of properly trained midwives have been eminently successful and of great advantage to the community. As proved by the evidence before your Committee, the services of midwives are a necessity . . .'

They referred to 'the apprehension expressed by certain witnesses belonging to the medical profession':

'Improved knowledge on the part of midwives will induce them to avail themselves more frequently and at an earlier stage than at present of skilled medical assistance in time of emergency and danger.'

If the Midwives' Institute were encouraged by that report, they could have received little cheer from the events that followed it. The battle became even more fierce, and a lay organisation was formed to carry it into wider fields – the Association for Promoting the Compulsory Registration of Midwives, in which prominent doctors and consultants joined with influential women in society and such bodies as the Women's Co-operative Guild, the National Union of Women Workers, and the Women's Liberal Federation. As part of its platform the Association included the representation of midwives on a Central Midwives' Board.

The Institute was grieved in February 1894 by the death of Mrs. Henry Smith. As Zepherina Veitch she had given it authority and strength from its foundation, and it was tragic that she did not live to see her great ambitions for the training and registration of midwives carried into effect. She was succeeded as president by Miss Jane Wilson, who as honorary secretary of the Workhouse Infirmary Nursing Association had devoted her life to the provision of trained nursing for the poorest of the community.

A ballot of the BMA on the subject of midwives' registration produced division: for example, Staffordshire, South Wales and Monmouth, Stirling, Kinross and Clackmannan were in favour, while the South Midlands, Cambridge and Huntingdonshire and West Somerset were against. More damaging was the success of a fight conducted at the General Medical Council by the implacable Dr. Rentoul and his supporters to have the diploma of the London Obstetrical Society outlawed. This must surely rank as one of the most petty and despicable acts. The diploma stated that its holder was 'a skilled midwife, competent to attend natural labour'. But the GMC, prodded by Dr. Rentoul, declared in December 1894 that the document was a 'colourable imitation' of a medical diploma.

The president of the London Obstetrical Society, who happened to be a leading champion of midwives, F.W. Champneys, agreed to re-word the diploma and to print it in a slightly smaller format. The examinations continued, and the diplomas were still awarded. But trained midwives were warned not to use the letters 'L.O.S.' after their names since some inno-

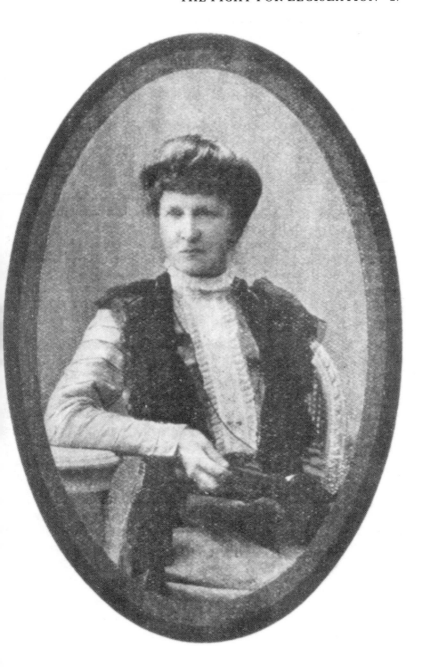

Miss Jane Wilson

cents – or less innocent and more determined doctors – were claiming that these letters represented not the 'London Obstetrical Society' but 'Licentiate of the Obstetrical Society', and that this must imply that the midwives were claiming to have a 'licence to practice' in rivalry to the medical profession.

It was nevertheless inevitable that the 'Midwives' Bill' would continue. In January 1895 a Midwives' Bill Committee met to draw up a further Bill. This time, medical interests were even more strongly represented since the Committee included the leading London obstetricians, as well as a representative of the Midwives' Institute (the president, Miss Wilson) and of the London Lying-in Hospital. The chairman was a leading Conservative peer, Lord Balfour of Burleigh. They produced a draft bill which was in some ways a regression, since examinations were to be conducted by local medical boards set up by the General Medical Council; and midwives were to be limited to attendance on 'natural labour'. There was to be no appeal to the Privy Council, and thus the GMC would have final authority over the scheme. The Midwives' Institute would have the right to nominate three members to a Central Midwives' Board, but they must all be doctors. Though far from happy at these developments, the Institute decided to support the proposed Bill 'from the standpoint of the public good'.

The Bill was introduced into the House of Lords by Lord Balfour on 18 May 1895, given its second reading, and sent to committee. At that point, it had been considerably redrafted. The examinations were to be controlled by a Central Midwives' Board and not by the GMC; the Board was to have three members appointed by the Crown to represent the public interest; and there was an additional and remarkable requirement that one of those Crown appointments must be a woman. The clause limiting a midwife's attendance to 'natural labour' was removed from the Bill, though it was to be incorporated in the supporting rules.

Evidently much work had been done behind the scenes. But it was nullified when in the same month the Government was defeated, and all pending legislation thus fell. Once again the drafters went to work, the BMA producing a draft which devalued the midwife to a 'midwifery nurse'.

There was certainly a gap between the trained midwife and the traditional 'neighbour woman', of whom Dickens' Sairey Gamp was the epitome of a bad example. Some doctors deliberately emphasised the class-barrier between the trained midwife and the local helper, for all her frequent imperfections. But the imperfections were many, and common sense dictated that training was necessary. As Sir William Priestley, doyen of obstetricians, remarked when opening the Liverpool Medical School in October 1896: 'Midwives should be properly educated, examined and then registered'. By that time, yet another Bill had appeared in the House of Commons (in May, and again in June) but had not been reached in the pressure of business.

Nursing Notes recorded that 'the President of the Midwives' Institute

Jane Wilson) was again asked to represent the Institute on the Midwives' Board Committee, and the Treasurer (Miss Paget) was also asked . . . The Midwives' Institute held a conference at the club in March when the Bill then brought before Parliament was read and discussed clause by clause'.

If the Bill did not move forward in the House, the Midwives' Institute was busily consolidating its position. In 1896, 128 new members joined; and the Institute began to organise midwifery training by districts, initially in London, but planning to extend the availability of training round the country.

The lay Association for Registration was also busy. A meeting was held at London House on 18 March, at which the chair was taken by Mrs. Creighton, wife of the Bishop of London. Her admirably clear, direct and lucid statement of aims deserves to be remembered:

'She said that what surprised her most was that there was any necessity for a meeting such as this in order to effect the registration of midwives. Their opponents did not take the trouble to understand what the Association had in view. It had been called a movement for the purpose of supplying the poor with midwives, but she failed to see why it had been so called. What they really wished to effect was that when a person sent for a midwife she should know that she got one, and not an untrained woman. Acts of Parliament had been passed to prevent people from being supplied with sand when they asked for sugar, and yet when a person sent for a nurse it was considered very criminal to desire to know whether the woman were qualified to call herself a midwife or not. Their opponents asserted that there was a design to turn the doctors out of the field, and also, on the other hand, to get rid of 'the friendly neighbour', but it was absolutely absurd to suppose that any Act of Parliament or registration could make it penal for one woman to help another in the moment of necessity. What they wished to prevent was that a person should deceive the public by assuming a position she was not intended to occupy. They wished that the examination for midwives should be as satisfactory as possible, their training as good as possible, and their registration in the hands of a competent authority.'

There now appeared on the scene a rival Bill. This was put forward by the British Medical Association, goaded and harassed by Dr Robert Rentoul. It was called the 'Obstetric Nurses' Registration Bill', and was intended to become 'An Act to provide for the Training, Compulsory Registration and Supervision of Midwifery Nurses'. The 'midwifery nurse' was defined as 'a woman who acts as a midwifery nurse in *all* cases of labour under the direct supervision of a medical practitioner at her confinement'. This proposal did not gain the support Rentoul expected and he shortly afterwards left the GMC.

Mrs Mary Nichol had resigned the secretaryship of the Midwives' Institute in 1897. She had served it devotedly during these years of challenge;

and her service was far from pompous for, a large and comfortable lady, she had an immense sense of humour and the accounts of those days are vivid with stories of the theatrical performances she would organise in the club. She delighted to tell the story of a cockney on top of a bus who, observing her generous proportions, asked: 'Tell me, mum, did you weigh heavy as a child?'

Her successor was Miss Paulina Fynes-Clinton, a trained midwife and close friend of Rosalind Paget. She had been a founder of the Institute, and for long a member of the Council. At this critical moment she took over its executive direction. It can have been no sinecure, for by this time there was a proliferation of committees – a Club Committee, and Educational Sub-Committee, a Midwives' Bill Sub-Committee and a Debates Sub-Committee. The Employment Register had now become an important part of the Institute's service, and was being used increasingly.

In February 1898 the Midwives' Bill was reintroduced into the House of Commons, this time by J.B. Balfour who as Lord Advocate for Scotland could summon legal opinion, and who had gained first place in the Private Members' ballot. The Bill was due for debate on 11 May; it transpired that the Government intended to take Private Members' time for Government legislation. A deputation was sent to the Lord President of the Council, the Duke of Devonshire, asking him to make the Bill a Government measure: he refused.

Meanwhile the Association for Promoting Compulsory Registration had lobbied the 244 coroners of England and Wales, as they were familiar with damage done by untrained midwives. They produced a list of 109 coroners who were willing to put their names to a recommendation for registration. However, the GMC had now adopted a hard line in respect of unqualified midwives, whom it wanted banned (despite the impracticability of this course: there were simply not enough qualified doctors and midwives to make this work). At this stage *Nursing Notes* aptly recorded that

'at the present moment a sort of triangular duel is going on between those who desire to see midwives under proper regulations, those who desire to see them suppressed, and those who pay a very strong respect to the liberty of the subject. It is impossible to please everybody . . .'

Jane Wilson resigned the presidency of the Midwives' Institute at the end of 1898, and Miss Amy Hughes was elected to succeed her. She was a 'Nightingale nurse', having been trained at St Thomas's. Then she had decided to choose district nursing, and trained with the Metropolitan and National Nursing Association (the predecessor of the Queen's Institute before working in Westminster and Chelsea. Later she became superintendent of the Central Home, and later at the Workhouse Hospital in Bolton Subsequently she became superintendent of the Nurse's Co-operation, then the largest body of private nurses.

The 'triangular duel' over registration went on into 1899, with the introduction of a further Midwives' Bill, again by J.B. Balfour.

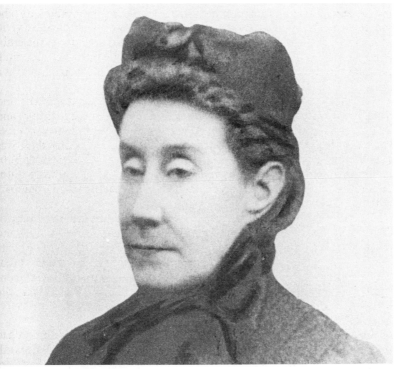

Miss Paulina Fynes-Clinton

Evidently it was impossible to please the midwives themselves; and *Nursing Notes* expressed itself with commendable restraint when in the summer of 1899 it recorded that

'The position of the Midwives' Institute with regard to the present Bill is not made easier by the attitude of The Manchester Midwives' Society, who would not sign a petition in its favour "in view of the objectionable features of the Bill which the Society has determined to oppose".'

The annoyance stemmed from the fact that the Manchester midwives had in fact been objecting to the Bill of 1898, and were a year behind the times. The new Bill, unsurprisingly, had various new features. It forbade unqualified midwives practising 'habitually and for gain', thus permitting a neighbour to give friendly help if required, provided she were not paid. It also contained a clause requiring midwives to produce references of good conduct, though holders of the London Obstetrical Society's diploma were to be exempt from it.

The influence of the Midwives' Institute by this time was so pervasive that the *British Medical Journal* took to referring to the Bill as 'the Bill of the Midwives' Institute', and Rosalind Paget wrote to the BMJ to refute this:

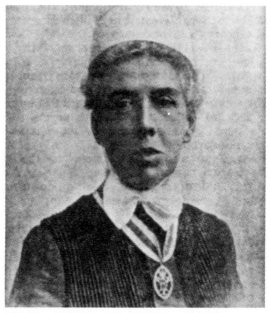

Miss Amy Hughes

'The Midwives' Institute have promoted no Bill since that introduced by Mr Fell Pease in 1890, in consequence of which the Committee on Midwives' Registration was appointed. From that time the Bill has been in more influential and competent hands than ours, and our part has been limited to sending a representative to the Bill Committee.'

It was, perhaps, in view of the powerful lobbying that the Institute had been conducting throughout, a somewhat ingenuous defence.

The 1889 Bill came up for debate on 12 April 1899, when again there was too little time and it was talked out. The events of the year were reported to the Institute in October at one of the periodical general meetings held at Buckingham Street, by Rosalind Paget.

Though successive bills leading to registration took up a great deal of the time and energy of the Institute's members in these years, this was not their only concern. For example, in June 1899 they voted to become affiliated to the Women's Institute, which had been founded two years earlier 'to supply the demand . . . for a centre of information and meeting place for those who are engaged in various departments of public, professional and philanthropic work, in science, literature and art.'

The Institute's committees had become more formalised. The Executive Council and Club Committee, consisting of ten members of Council and ten members of the Club, met on the second Friday in the month at 8 o'clock. Other committees were the Educational Committee, comprising the lecturers on midwifery, monthly nursing, hygiene, the class teacher, the treasurer and secretary; the Sectional Committee on Midwifery (twenty-two vice-presidents and members of Council, all midwives); the Sectional Committee on Nursing (twenty-two members, all trained nurses); and the Debates Sub-Committee (chaired by the President, with an honorary secretary and four members).

At last in 1899 it seemed that the Midwives' Bill stood some reasonable chance of success within a few years. In that July the Lord President of the Council, the Duke of Devonshire, responded more positively to a deputation:

'I should suggest that you should make use of this department [the Privy Council] . . . as the means of communication with those authorities whose support it is necessary for you to enlist, namely the medical profession and the county authorities.'

This was indeed a breakthrough, if the Privy Council was to be the focal point to bring the midwives to a consensus with the medical bodies and the local authorities (particularly the latter, since the Local Government Board had throughout the previous decade refused to become involved).

The draft Bill of 1900 was introduced by Mr Heywood Johnstone, given a second reading, sent to the Grand Committee on Law – and then talked out. In 1901 the Bill did not reappear at all, since its potential sponsors were unsuccessful in the Private Members' ballot. In 1902, though, they were successful and the latest version of the Bill was put forward for its second reading on 26 February. This time there was a most material change in its provisions, for the proposed Central Midwives' Board was to be independent of the General Medical Council, and instead directly responsible to the Privy Council. The Bill was introduced by Lord Cecil Manners, supported by Mr A. de Tatton Egerton (who had put forward the Bill of 1896), who was chairman of the General Lying-in Hospital.

The Bill was discussed by the Standing Committee of the House in March. Vigorous attempts by some medical M.P.s to have the representation of Midwives' Institute removed from the proposed Midwives' Board did not succeed. When the Bill came to its report stage in the House on 6 June, the Home Secretary said that he could not support a Bill that would immediately outlaw all untrained midwives, and thus leave some areas of the country without midwifery aid. It was suggested that a date might be set at which unqualified midwives would have to register or cease to practice: the year 1910, eight years away, was suggested, and this was agreed by Mr Heywood Johnstone on behalf of the sponsors. The opposition then largely disappeared, though in the confusion the Royal British Nurses' Association was provided with representation on the Central Midwives' Board (while ironically at that stage the Queen's Institute was unrepresented, an anomaly that was hastily to be repaired later).

The Midwives' Bill received its third reading from both Houses on 2 July, and the Royal Assent was given on 31 July 1902. In *Nursing Notes* for September 1902 Rosalind Paget wrote a long survey of twenty years of endeavour. It is a fair and, in the circumstances, a most restrained account, though understandably she did not undervalue the work done by the Midwives' Institute. Though the Midwives' Act (as it now, at last, became) was a compromise, and applied only to England and Wales (and not Scotland or Ireland), 'the factors that have been concerned in the result attained are by no means so few or so easily recognised as is sometimes thought'.

She referred to the three interested parties: the public, the medical profession and the midwife:

'We can very shortly deal with the attitude of the midwives. The trained ones have always been favourable to some legislation, for exceedingly simple reasons, the following being chief among them: (1) that after spending money and time in qualifying themselves in the best way possible for their work, they had no status; and (2) that any woman, however ignorant and incapable, has been allowed to call herself a midwife, and practise. Naturally as the trained midwife is in a minority, the doings of these untrained women disgraced the whole body. None knew better than the trained midwife how serious is the state of things, and they have always asked at least for some protection of the word "midwife". The untrained midwives, many of whom may have been most worthy, and from long experience and help from the doctors, doubtless in their way very competent, have made no demand for legislation.'

Rosalind Paget described at length the strongly held views of the various groups of the medical profession. Then she turned to the Act itself, and picked out certain clauses for comment.

Clause 1(1) protected the title of midwife:

'From and after the first day of April 1905, any woman who not being certified under this Act shall take or use the name or title of midwife (either alone or in combination with any other word or words), or any name, title, addition, or description implying that she is certified under this Act, or is a person specially qualified to practice midwifery, or is recognised by law as a midwife, shall be liable on summary conviction to a fine not exceeding five pounds.'

Clause 1(2) concerned 'practice for gain', and laid down that after 1 April 1910 'no woman shall habitually and for gain attend women in childbirth otherwise than under the direction of a qualified medical practitioner unless she be certified under this Act'. The words about the 'direction of a qualified medical practitioner' were intended to safeguard the 'monthly nurse'; but, as Miss Paget pointed out, the clause did imply the right of qualified midwives to work independently of a doctor.

Clause 1(4) stated that 'No woman certified under this Act shall employ an uncertified person as her substitute'; the Institute had established that this would not interfere with the education of pupils.

Clause 1(5) was inserted, wrote Miss Paget, 'to make the medical practitioner happy. It stated:

'The certificate under this Act shall not confer upon any woman any right or title to be registered under the Medical Acts or to assume any name, title, or designation implying that she is by law recognised as a medical practitioner, or that she is authorised to grant any medical certificate, or any certificate of death or of still-birth, or to undertake the charge of cases of abnormality or disease in connection with parturition.'

This was 'of no consequence whatever to the trained midwife', said Miss Paget.

There was at this time no legal requirement that still-births should be registered, and any citizen had the right to 'declare' a death. It was therefore important that midwives present at a still-birth should record it by beginning 'I declare . . .' and not 'I certify . . .' Of such details are laws made.

Two more important matters about which Miss Paget chose to comment were the means whereby practising midwives, trained and untrained, were to be brought within the Act; and secondly, the composition of the Central Midwives' Board.

The relevant clause to govern the transition from an unregulated to a regulated profession read:

'Any woman who, within two years from the date of this Act coming into operation, claims to be certified under this Act, shall be so certified provided she holds a certificate in midwifery from the Royal College of Physicians of Ireland, or from the Obstetrical Society of London, or the Coombe Lying-in Hospital and Guinness's Dispensary, or the Rotunda Hospital for the Relief of the Poor Lying-in Women of Dublin, or such other certificate as may be approved by the Central Midwives' Board, or produces evidence, satisfactory to the Board, that at the passing of this Act, she had been for at least one year in *bona fide* practice as a midwife and that she bears a good character.'

The last phrase was contentious, since it referred to the general character of the midwife and not her professional character, and so unlike any other professional qualification it widened the question of 'character' to cover personal and private life. Miss Paget made no comment on it, however.

She dealt at length with the duties of the local supervising authority, which was to be the County or Borough Council; and she noted that the one emergency in which those authorities might act without reference upwards was to prevent the spread of infection.

The relevant clause empowered them 'to suspend any midwife from practice . . . if such suspension appears necessary, *in order to prevent the spread of infection*'. Extraordinarily, this last sub-clause was deleted from the Bill in the House of Commons, thus laying midwives open to local suspension for any reason that the local authority thought fit. At the behest of the Midwives' Institute, the sub-clause was restored in the House of Lords.

Finally, Miss Paget considered the composition of the Central Midwives' Board. It was to consist of four registered medical practitioners, appointed one each by the Royal College of Physicians, the Royal College of Surgeons, the Society of Apothecaries, and the Midwives' Institute. Two persons (one a woman) were to be appointed by the Lord President of the Privy Council; and one each by the Association of County Councils, Queen Victoria's Jubilee Institute, and the Royal British Nurses' Association.

There was thus no direct requirement that a qualified midwife should sit on the Central Midwives' Board. Miss Paget was prepared to accept this. 'True, we can only appoint a medical practitioner, but the matters that will arise are sure to be both medical and technical, and I can imagine we are more likely to have our case put with weight by a doctor who can meet others of the same profession on their own ground than by any midwife, however able'.

The Board was important, since 'it makes rules and regulations for the issue of certificates, for training examination, for supervision, restrictions, suspension, removal from the roll etc. It is the central authority for carrying out the provisions of the Act.'

At a special meeting of the Midwives' Institute held at Buckingham Street on 17 October 1902, Dr Charles James Cullingworth was invited to be the first representative of the Institute on the Central Midwives' Board. He accepted. At the same meeting, in a most felicitous gesture, it was agreed on the proposal of Dr. Annie McCall that a message of congratulation be sent to Louisa Hubbard, lying ill in Austria, on the successful completion of a work to which she had set her hand a quarter of a century before.

The Privy Council was able to announce the composition of the first Central Midwives' Board. As *Nursing Notes* commented in some amazement, 'It is the unexpected that always happens, and if we had been requested to forecast the composition of this Board it would certainly not have been the present one.'

Royal College of Physicians: Dr Champneys
Royal College of Surgeons: Mr Ward Cousins (Portsmouth)
Society of Apothecaries: Dr Parker Young (Westbourne Square)
Incorporated Midwives' Institute: Dr Cullingworth
Privy Council: Dr Sinclair (Manchester)
                Miss Jane Wilson
Association of County Councils: Mr Heywood Johnstone Esq. M.P.
Queen Victoria's Jubilee Institute for Nurses: Miss R. Paget
Royal British Nurses' Association: Miss Oldham

There were six men and three women. 'When we look at important bodies such as Parliament, County Councils, and Borough Councils, where no woman can sit' (said *Nursing Notes*), and at the proportion of women to men on the School Board, Boards of Guardians etc., we cannot but think the proportion of women on this Board is satisfactory, and that women a.

women may be fairly satisfied.'

In Dr Champneys and Dr Cullingworth the Institute had two of its staunchest supporters who between them spanned a wide range of experience. Of the medical men, 'two are eminent consultants . . . one is a general practitioner, another a most representative medical man from the north of England, and the fifth is from the south of England and has had largely to do with the British Medical Association. Heywood Johnstone M.P. had piloted the 1902 Bill through the House of Commons. All three of the women on the Board were trained midwives; Jane Wilson a past president of the Midwives' Institute, Rosalind Paget its treasurer though sitting as representative of the Queen's Institute, as a member of its Council. Miss Oldham, a member of the Council of the Royal British Nurses' Association, was also a long-time member of the Midwives' Institute.

Nursing Notes remarked:

'It is one of life's little ironies that these three women should be prominent members of the Midwives' Institute whose representation at all on the Central Board has been so much debated and has constantly hung in the balance. The midwives, we think, need not fear that their interests will for the future be ignored'.

Now it was up to the midwives. Rosalind Paget had rubbed the message in:

'To sum up, trained midwives, now that you are recognised by Act of Parliament, what body of workers have you to thank that you are not by law called midwifery or obstetric nurses? That your vested rights in your certificates of training have been considered? That you have a representative on the governing body? That you are not bound hand and foot under those who have only too openly shown how they would 'end' you if only they had the power? Who has worked, unflinchingly, through the hard years of indifference, contempt, suspicion, to a modicum of consideration and respect in order to create for you a respected and worthy status?

I am writing in my own person and under my own name and therefore I take this opportunity of telling you that you owe all this and much more to the Council of the Incorporated Midwives' Institute. No one not of this Council knows how difficult has been that work, how discouraging, and how when our motives were misrepresented we were obliged to 'refrain even from good words though it was pain and grief to us'.

Are you going to let this work be lost, are you going to let your heritage lapse for want of a little energy? Those of us who have worked this question are no longer young, and we are very tired; but we can put the younger ones in the way of organising their profession if they will come to us and take advantage of our long and weary experience, and we will then thankfully sing our 'Nunc Dimittis'.

The first meeting of the Central Midwives' Board was convened at the

Privy Council office on 11 December 1902. All members attended, Dr F.H. Champneys was chosen as chairman, a post he was to occupy for twenty-seven years. Sir Francis Champneys – he was knighted in 1909 – was an excellent choice. Obstetrical physician at St George's Hospital and the General Lying-in Hospital, York Road, he had been a member of the London Obstetrical Society examining board from 1882, chairman from 1891–95, and president of the Society in 1895. He had been educated at Winchester and Oxford, and then became a medical student at Bart's. As a young man he had spent half a year each on travelling scholarships in Vienna, Leipzig and Dresden, and was thus well aware of the more effective European regulation of midwives.

His background and experience was in pleasant contrast to that of the representative of the Midwives' Institute on the Board – Dr Charles James Cullingworth. His professional career had largely been spent in the north of England, at Leeds and then at Manchester, where he became lecturer in medical jurisprudence at Owen's College (the antecedent of Manchester University) in 1879, attaining the chair of Obstetrics and Gynaecology in 1885, which he was to hold for nineteen years although from 1888 he also worked in London as obstetrical physician at St Thomas's Hospital.

Between them, Champneys and Cullingworth spanned a wide range of experience, and they were united in their assurance that the work of the Board was necessary and urgent. Their work was strengthened by the presence as representative of the Local Government Board of Heywood Johnstone, whose enthusiasm for the work was no less than theirs, and whose presence was an indication that the local authorities would be persuaded to make the scheme work.

In May 1903 the Local Government Board issued a memorandum to county councils and town councils of county boroughs 'with reference to the provisions of the Midwives' Act 1902'. The Act had technically come into force in April 1903, but no rules had then been promulgated and the local authorities were thrown into some confusion as they tried to work out how it should be interpreted. Northamptonshire, for example, issued a formidable poster warning all women who used the title of 'Midwife' that they would be affected by the Act and must communicate with the Medical Officer of Health.

Bradford Corporation delegated authority to its Health Committee, Gloucestershire to its Sanitary Committee, Northamptonshire (eventually) to its Public Health Committee. West Suffolk got into an impasse: *Nursing Notes* reported that 'the Committee seemed to consider that their powers should be delegated to the Urban District Council of Bury St Edmunds at present. So far as we can gather from the report the Urban District Council of Bury St Edmunds did not agree, so the matter was referred back'. This was marginally better than the performance in Newcastle City Council, where 'Mr Alfred Appleby asked a series of questions dealing with the new Midwives Act, 1902, whereat the assembled members laughed heartily and the town clerk replied.'

By the summer of 1903 the Central Midwives' Board had its own offices at 6 Suffolk Street, Pall Mall, and a permanent secretary, G.W. Duncan. The rules were drafted, approved by the Privy Council on 12 August, and printed. They included 'suggestions to County and County Borough Councils as to the working of the Act and the delegation of powers', which somewhat ameliorated the confusion.

No. _1_   .Date _Oct 29th 1903_

Central Midwives Board.

(2 Edw. VII. ch. 17.)

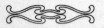

We hereby Certify

That _Mary Ann Eleanor Stephens_

is entitled by law to practise as a Midwife in accordance

with the provisions of the Midwives Act, 1902, and subject

to the rules and regulations laid down in pursuance

thereof, by virtue of having been in *bonâ fide* practice as

a Midwife for one year prior to the 31st July, 1902.

F. H. Champney, M.D. ⎫ Members
Chas. J. Cullingworth M.D. ⎬ of the
                            ⎭ Board.
G. W. Duncan Secretary.

The first certificate issued by the Central Midwives' Board, to Mrs Mary Ann Stephens in 1902

TWO

Enrolment and Education

The Midwives' Roll was opened by the Central Midwives' Board on 29 October 1903. The first name inscribed upon it was that of Mrs Mary Ann Stephens. This represented a generous and sensitive act by Rosalind Paget, whose name might well have come first as a tribute to the relentless hard work she had put into the campaign. But it was typical of her that she gave the honour of being Britain's first enrolled midwife to the 'senior member' of the Midwives' Institute who for twenty-one years was a practising midwife in Tottenham, and who by her death seven years later had delivered over 8,000 infants.

Mary Ann Eleanor Stephens had trained at the City of London Lying-in Hospital, and taken the LOS Diploma in 1881. She fully supported the aims of the Midwives' Institute and when its 'founders' prospectus' was being drawn up, hers was the first name upon it. (Her certificate, together with those of the next three enrolments, now hangs in the library of the Royal College of Midwives.) She lost no opportunity to widen her knowledge, and held the gold medal for first aid of the St John Ambulance Association. It was said of her that 'her common sense, which was always combined with kindness, together with her great practical experience of midwifery, made her opinions of great advantage to, and much considered by, the younger members of the profession because . . . Mrs Stephens was an exceedingly successful midwife, popular in her district, both with patients and with doctors, who always seemed willing to go to her in any difficulty because she would always go and do odd jobs for them'.

Her down-to-earth manner is illustrated by one contribution she made to a discussion at the Midwives' Institute, when at a time of strong feelings about the demarcation of duties she was asked whether the midwife should be obliged to wash the baby. 'It may be *infra dig*,' said Mrs Stephens, 'but it would be exceedingly *heartless* not to wash the poor baby.' Her kindness kept her sometimes short of money: she would 'forget' to take fees from poor patients, and her son recalled touchingly that at 'Sunday's dinner at home, the prime cut from the joint was always for some poor deserving patient'. She was an excellent choice to epitomise the best of the practising midwives of her time, and very fit to take first place on the Midwives' Roll. Second place went to Rosalind Paget, third place to the secretary of the Institute, Paulina Fynes-Clinton, and fourth to Amy Hughes, a future president.

Once the aim of registration had been achieved, the Midwives' Institute set itself to the next task, to devise an adequate and nationally available system of training. The requirement under the newly-published Rules was modest indeed: a midwife must have three months' training, in the official view. Training therefore became a major activity of the next few years. The examination of the London Obstetrical Society ceased, and was replaced by a not dissimilar examination conducted by the Central Midwives' Board, to be held four times a year (Rosalind Paget thought that an inadequate provision, and was proved right).

Despite its leaders' endeavours in travelling round the country to speak to provincial groups and conferences, the Institute was still a metropolitan and not a national organisation. All its 'centres' were in London, except for one in Cambridge.

The friends of the Institute rallied to this new cause. The Association for the Compulsory Registration of Midwives, having accomplished its task, did not disband but transformed itself under the secretaryship of Mrs Heywood Johnstone into the Association for Promoting the Training and Supply of Midwives. Its chairman was the Archbishop of Canterbury (and three years later Queen Alexandra became its Patron).

But no one knew for certain the scale of the problem, since before registration there was no sure way of discovering how many women in the country were practising as midwives. A decade earlier, a census estimate was 3,000; but Dr Aveling had believed that many would not have identified themselves as such in a census, and that the true number must be around 9,000. It was now law that midwives must enrol, either as 'trained' midwives or as 'bona fide' midwives, by 1 April 1905. When the Roll was made up on that date, it demonstrated that even Aveling had substantially underestimated. The Roll contained 22,308 names, of whom 7,465 were certificated by the London Obstetrical Society, 2,322 had hospital certificates, and 12,521 were uncertificated midwives in bona fide practice. While these figures were illuminating, they were distorted by the fact that a number of trained nurses who had taken a midwifery qualification were not practising midwives also enrolled.

The Association for Promoting the Training and Supply of Midwives took speedy action to provide training, opening a training school 'in cooperation with the Plaistow Maternity Charity at East Ham', where four pupils could take a sixteen-week course (at a cost of £19.6s.8d. including board); in three years, forty-one midwives took the course and passed the LOS diploma exam.

The Association also sponsored training vacancies at several London hospitals and at Glasgow and Cheltenham. The Institute organised its own courses consisting of twenty-six lectures, four times a year; and an 'anonymous donor' provided £200 a year for three years, to support training. The running battle with some of the representatives of the medical profession continued; in 1904 the British Gynaecological Society issued a statement that 'the Midwives' Act has created a sharp line of division between those who desire to be registered as midwives, that is to say, who desire to work as independent practitioners, under the Midwives' Board, and for the most part among the very poor, and those who desire to do maternity nursing under the supervision of medical practitioners, and, for the most part, among the middle and upper classes . . . The nurse who becomes registered as a midwife obtains a definite legal status as a practitioner of midwifery; but on the other hand, she is not likely to receive any assistance or work from medical practitioners as a monthly nurse.'

Some doctors continued to take this hard line for a number of years; and from time to time the matter was aired at inquests when doctors had refused to answer the call of an enrolled midwife. However, the doctors who carried their opposition to such an extreme were fortunately few, and became fewer as the effectiveness of the trained midwife became apparent.

A large number of doctors did see a threat in the further medical education of midwives. When in March 1901 the Institute announced a 'postgraduate lecture' (it was by Dr Eden, on haemorrhage), there were medical objections that midwives were not 'graduates' and so were not entitled to use the term 'postgraduate'; the title was dropped.

By this time medical lectures were a feature of the Institute's calendar, and well attended. In 1904 the Institute's officers were drawing up plans for monthly lectures and short courses for 'bona fide' midwives.

The five-year 'period of grace' between 1905 and 1910 was intended as a reasonable time in which the old generation of unlettered midwives would give way to the new. It did not happen like that, not least because the congested urban centres of population, the overcrowded cities, depended to a great extent on the midwife of folklore. Nor were the local authorities eager to accept their statutory responsibilities: the London County Council at first proposed to delegate its monitoring powers to its constituent councils, and it took a strong protest by the Midwives' Institute to persuade the LCC to exercise those powers itself. However, once that had been agreed, the LCC worked positively, organising training courses for midwives.

The Central Midwives' Board was early faced with the problem of the fair and reasonable way of dealing with the bona fide midwives brought before them for incompetence. The plain fact was that many of these women had been 'practising' by native wit for many years; while the good ones might be very good indeed, the bad ones inflicted terrible carnage. In July 1905 the Board struck off five of them for breaking the rules. One 'could not read or write, could not use a clinical thermometer, and did not know what a catheter was'. The Board had some sympathy with her, and 'thought that it was more her misfortune than her fault that this action was necessary. The Board had, however, to carry out the Act as it stood and . . . the safety of the lying-in woman was its first care'.

As the catalogue of tragedy and ignorance unfolded at meeting after meeting of the Central Midwives' Board the Midwives' Institute made determined efforts to encourage practising women to become trained. *Nursing Notes* (which from 1908 added '*and Midwives' Chronicle*' to its title, thus regularising what had already been apparent) noted with approval that, for example, in Mansfield, Nottinghamshire, fifty-four midwives from the neighbourhood had been invited to attend lectures, and thirty-eight had taken the trouble to do so. As editor of *Nursing Notes*, Emma Brierly made a brave effort to widen her readership by reporting news of practising midwives whether trained or untrained; thus in 1910 she noted the death of Mrs Elizabeth Green of Cardiff at the age of ninety-one. Mrs Green had practised up to the age of 80, having attended over 4,000 cases, of whom only one died.

From 1905 the Midwives' Institute was planning courses of instruction for pupil midwives, with two lectures a week and an examination at the end of three months. Post graduate lectures were also started for those midwives training pupils on the district.

During the five years of the 'period of grace' the positive effects of the Midwives' Act and its potential for good gradually became apparent. Inspectors had been appointed by most local authorities. In his annual report for 1906 the County Medical Officer for Wiltshire wrote:

'The Midwives' Act has been spoken of . . . as a useless, absurd and altogether unworkable Act, that will be productive of no good. My experience leads me to quite the contrary opinion . . . I consider it entirely workable . . . and can be converted into a most valuable Act that will be the means of lessening much suffering, and saving the lives of many mothers and children.'

Dr Merry Smith, the LCC's inspector, went further. Speaking to a conference on infant mortality he said:

'It is obvious that, as women trained under the Act take the place of the illiterate, incompetent persons that very generally look after the poor at this critical period of their lives, a great opportunity is offered for giving mothers the information wanted and providing the newly-born infant with a fair start.'

The Midwives' Institute inevitably became the focal point for information about the Act and its workings, and this duty was eagerly taken up. In one of her treasurer's reports, Rosalind Paget looked back to the days, only a few years before, when the Institute had a club-room open once a week from 6 till 10, a very small library, and a secretary who answered letters and attended once a week (Mrs Nichol).

'Think what a difference now! Seven rooms, an Organising Secretary and an Assistant Secretary, lectures, Midwives in Council [this was a periodic discussion meeting], a perfectly superb medical lending library, light literature, and medical and nursing papers; a representative on the Central Midwives' Board, a Council consisting entirely of experts in the midwifery profession, and a special Midwives' Advisory Committee to look after your interests with the Central Midwives' Board, and all this for the same sum of 5s. a year. I really don't know how we manage it.'

As 1910 approached, the midwives in the country began to realise that not only was the Act working, but that from 1 April 1910 no midwife would be legally permitted to practise unless she were enrolled. Associations began to spring up all over the country, notably a Midwives' Defence Union. The officers of the Midwives' Institute toured the country, explaining the advantages of a single united voice. By 1909 there were associations of midwives in Northumberland, Durham, Liverpool, Bolton, Hull, Cardiff, Gloucester, Swansea, Newport, Ipswich, Hertfordshire, and Sussex, as well as sixteen separate associations in London. One by one they were persuaded to affiliate to the Institute, until by 1910 there were thirty-five affiliated associations.

A Departmental Committee was set up to consider the working of the Act. The chairman of the Central Midwives' Board, Sir Francis Champneys, was recruited; but there was no midwife on the Committee. This extraordinary omission so outraged Jane Wilson that she resigned from the Central Midwives' Board in protest. Her protest – which as she was president, was effectively that of the Institute – was received with the customary and polite expressions of regret, but nothing was done about it. When the Departmental Committee reported, it was with the bland opinion that 'no shortage of midwives need be anticipated, the difficulty being mainly one of distribution'.

Jane Wilson was worried that the interests of midwives would be overlooked or ignored by the law-makers. Parliament was entirely male, and women did not then have the vote (and did not achieve it until 1918, and then only at the age of thirty; in 1928 they were given the vote at twenty-one). The demand for female suffrage was growing, and was being expressed in the sometimes violently militant activities of the Suffragettes. The Midwives' Institute supported the demand for women to have the vote, though reproving militant demonstrations. Nevertheless some midwives became active suffragettes, and one at least went to gaol for her activities. The Central Midwives' Board took a remarkably liberal view when they received a report from the Governor of Holloway Prison that a midwife had been taken there, having been convicted of 'damaging government property'. Although according to the rules she should have been immediately and automatically struck off the Roll, having committed a criminal offence, the Board allowed the letter to 'lie on the table', taking no action upon it, because her offence had been 'political'.

Miss Wilson's fears were confirmed when in May 1910 the Government published a second Midwives' Bill. It proposed that a representative of the British Medical Association should be added to the Board, together with representatives of the administering authorities – the Local Government Board, the Association of Municipal Corporations, and the Society of Medical Officers of Health. At last, it was proposed that there should be two certified midwives on the Board as representatives of the Midwives' Institute and the Royal British Nurses' Association (there had been three certified midwives on the Board at its foundation, but this had been by the accident of nomination, and not by legal requirement).

The Famous Four (Amy Hughes, Jane Wilson, Rosalind Paget and Paulina Fynes-Clinton) fought back strongly.

'We would ask that it should be laid down in the Act that the lying-in woman shall have entirely free choice as to whether she employs a doctor or a midwife, and liberty to choose that doctor or midwife; also, if she employs a midwife, and it is necessary for the midwife to send for a doctor, that his fee shall be assured. The medical profession is able through its powerful organisations to influence Parliament. The midwife is, by reason of her sex, excluded from any participation in making the laws that concern her, and the only hope of obtaining a small modicum of justice is by appealing to the public through the Press.'

They wrote innumerable letters. They addressed meetings. They lobbied MPs and argued with doctors and administrators. A Committee on the position of women under the National Insurance Bill sat at the House of Commons, and Rosalind Paget addressed it. She also went to see David Lloyd George, being as she said 'representative of the Incorporated Midwives' Institute and its 35 affiliated associations, and of the 32,000 midwives on the Midwives' Roll'.

That autumn in Parliament a clause was added to the National Insurance Bill that

'the mother shall decide whether she shall be attended by a registered medical practitioner or by a duly certified midwife, and shall have free choice in the selection of such practitioner or midwife.'

The 30s. (£1.50p) maternity benefit could therefore be paid either to a doctor or midwife; and though arguments followed concerning payment when a midwife called in a doctor, the principle was established in law.

The sturdy independence of the midwife up and down the country had scarcely been affected by the new legislation. In the first year of enrolment, 1905, a startling situation had come to light in rural districts. Of the 519 London midwives on the Roll in that year, the great majority (318) were trained. But in Durham, of 264 enrolled midwives only 51, or one fifth, were trained. And in the whole of the county of Norfolk, only 70 midwives were enrolled, of whom a mere 10 were trained.

By 1910 the position had improved somewhat (2,281 midwives passed the Board examination in that year alone); but of 103 disciplinary cases reported to the Board that year, 60 were struck off the Roll for malpractice; and a further 88 'midwives' voluntarily removed their names that year. Nevertheless, despite the view of the Departmental Committee that there was no shortage of midwives, the Board enrolled a further 515 bona fide (untrained) midwives that year on the recommendation of local authorities, who feared just such a shortage. The Midwives Institute thought this enrolment of untrained women 'deplorable'.

The increase in the number of trained midwives might be expected to have had some influence on infant mortality, and indeed it did. This was general throughout the country, though particularly marked in London, where there were 160 deaths per 1,000 in 1900, and 106 per thousand in 1910. Durham showed less impact (167 per thousand to 128 per thousand), though Norfolk showed a remarkable improvement (142 per thousand to 84 per thousand).

Matters were therefore improving, and the increase in the number of trained midwives could be adduced as one of the causes of this improvement. The Midwives' Institute could reasonably claim to have been mainly responsible for the determined campaigning that had brought this about. The authority of the Institute was now acknowledged in government, and among administrators: when the newly-formed Association of Inspectors of Midwives held its first meeting in September 1910 it was at the Midwives' Institute in Buckingham Street.

Yet the country's midwives did not join the Institute, and the circulation of *Nursing Notes and the Midwives' Chronicle* remained small, and the journal itself an uncommercial drain on its editor's pocket. This apathy to association among the majority of midwives irritated Rosalind Paget, who in May 1915 wrote an open letter to practising midwives in the columns of *Nursing Notes*. It was headlined WAKE UP, MIDWIVES!

'You live such isolated, as well as such very busy and anxious lives that you do not seem to hear of what is going on in the world around you or if you do, you do not realise its importance to yourself – and your profession . . . Now if you will not read the journal that has consistently voiced your interests for twenty-seven years, nor support the Institute that was incorporated in 1890 to improve your status and protect your rights, you cannot expect that Institute to continue to work for you without any support as it has done in the past, or continue the thankless task of fighting for the rights of a body of women who still, after all these years, seem to take no interest whatever in the organisation of their own profession. I speak plainly, but the time has come for it.

You have had in the past certain chances of showing that you are a profession of intelligent women who intend to make their voice heard in matters that concern their own work. The first good opportunity you had was when the Midwives' Act was passed: you did not take it, but left it entirely to the Midwives' Institute and the handful of intelligent women of which it was then composed to fight for your rights and insist on justice under that Act. They secured you your representative on the Central Midwives' Board, but how many of you care in the least who that representative is or what is done by the representative? At that time, if it had not been for the Midwives' Institute you would have found yourselves with the word "midwife" unprotected, with no representation on the Board that governs you and makes rules and regulations for you . . .

The second good opportunity you had was when the Insurance Bill was passed. By that time I am glad to say the Midwives' Institute was in a stronger position, owing chiefly to the large number of associations of midwives in the country that had affiliated to the central body, and they were able to obtain the insertion of the word "midwife" into the Act, and, further, that the mother should have free choice of whether she employed a doctor or a midwife: if this had not been done you would have been entirely wiped off the face of the earth and it would have been no use for anyone to have been a midwife. Though you surely knew all this, you have not supported those who obtained these concessions for you. You are willing to benefit by all that is done for your profession without making any effort to cooperate with them.'

This strong appeal was published in the columns of *Nursing Notes*, which meant of course that it was read only by those who subscribed to the journal and so were not those apathetic people whom Rosalind Paget was addressing. It is, of course, the perpetual complaint of the activists in every walk of life who, concerning themselves passionately with some movement, cannot understand why those less perceptive than themselves are so careless of their rights and responsibilities. No one had more justification than Rosalind Paget to write in this way; and probably no one was less surprised than she when change continued to happen in its familiar slow, bumbling British fashion. If the midwives listened, they acted slowly, slowly.

The particular cause of her outburst was the publication of a circular by the Local Government Board on maternity and child welfare. It was a scheme to improve the health of mother and child before, during and after childbirth, but once again it did not place any particular weight on the possible influence of the midwife.

'The questions at issue are very serious and are not generally grasped by the philanthropic public (wrote Rosalind Paget). We midwives know that there is a great deal of abortion that might be prevented: we wish to help to prevent this. We are in a position to recognise certain constitutional diseases that ought to be referred to a medical practitioner for treatment: we also recognise the importance of seeing that this treatment is properly carried out. I cannot help feeling that we ought to be very willing to cooperate in this crusade . . . But if our honest cooperation is given, those organising the schemes must understand what the position of the midwife is: she is in charge of the patient from the time she books until ten days after the labour, and during that time the midwife is the person to say if her patient requires medical attention; she is trained to do this in a way that health visitors and other workers are not . . . We should make careful investigation of our cases, and if in the certain number that will require medical treatment either for some threatened accident or constitutional disease, we can get into touch with the maternity and child welfare organisation, some good may be done, if, however, we set ourselves like a blank wall against all this and say that our patients shall not have anything to do with these centres, if we set our patients against these organisations, which of course we can very well do, we shall be acting in an exceedingly short-sighted manner and one which in the end will react upon ourselves. We are not a strong trades union, like the medical profession, we shall simply be brushed aside, our exceedingly valuable help will be ignored, as it often has been in the past, our patients will be interfered with by amateurs with no special knowledge of the subject, they will be taken away from us and we shall in the future become of no account whatever, and this, may I say, we shall richly deserve.'

During the fifty years that followed, the health services were to be increasingly centralised and organised by the State. Rosalind Paget saw the future very clearly, saw the dangers of refusing to play an active part in the control of the new systems, and chivvied the midwives into positive participation. In October 1915 the Midwives' Institute launched its first course of lectures at Buckingham Street on what was then called 'Ante-natal Care', including lectures on the influence of the environment, on venereal disease, and on abortion.

The Midwives' Act of 1902 did not apply to Scotland. For once, and most unusually, Scottish law was behind English; and it was not until 1916 that a Midwives Act was introduced for Scotland. When it was, it introduced various provisions that had been discussed as improvements for the English Act in 1911, but not yet introduced. There was to be a separate Central Midwives' Board for Scotland, which had the power (which the English Board did not) to suspend midwives breaking the rules: the English Board could only strike them from the Roll. However, the Scottish Act included the controversial phrase that allowed women to practise as midwives provided they did not do so 'habitually and for gain'; but it did allow the midwives' expenses to be paid, and made provision for a doctor's fee to be paid when sent for by a midwife. When the Scottish Board was set up, however, no midwives were included upon it, though Lady Balfour of Burleigh and Lady Susan Gilmour were members, and both were acknowledged to be well informed on the conditions under which midwives and nurses worked.

During the setting up of the Central Midwives' Board for Scotland there was much correspondence between Scottish midwives and the Midwives' Institute in London. Soon after the Act was passed one of the Scottish midwives, Mrs Quintin Smith of Lanarkshire, organised her fellow midwives into the Scottish Midwives Association, of which she was appointed Honorary Secretary, a post she was to hold for twenty-five years. A Constitution was drawn up and gradually branches were formed throughout Scotland.

The passing of the Scottish Act introduced an odd anomaly. For the

Scottish Act empowered English midwives to practise in Scotland, but because the English Midwives' Act of 1902 did not apply to Scotland, and because no one at that time thought of putting in a reciprocity clause, Scottish midwives could not practise in England. This situation prevailed for a further two years, while the Midwives' Institute lobbied continually for an Amending Act to bring the English provisions into line with the more enlightened Scottish arrangements.

As the Great War drew towards its end, legislation was introduced. The Bill received its third reading on 31 October and the second Midwives' Act came into operation on 1 January 1919.

It was sad that the secretary of the Midwives' Institute, Paulina Fynes-Clinton, did not live to see it, for she died on 16 September. In her quiet and self-effacing way she had done much to establish the status of the midwife. She was a trained nurse, once a Sister at the London Hospital and for three years Assistant Matron. Her midwifery training was at Endell Street; she had joined the Midwives' Institute in 1886 and was a signatory of the Articles of Association in 1889. She was a member of the Institute Council to her death. She was also a trained masseuse, and a founder of the Incorporated Society of Trained Masseuses. One of her most valuable activities was the supervision of midwifery training, and for some years she organised and taught the training courses held at the Institute. For a period she also acted as a visitor to the nurses of the Workhouse Nursing Association; her slogan was 'the best for the poorest'. She never had the flamboyance of her close friend Rosalind Paget, but by her dedication and care ensured the smooth running of the Institute in a time of challenge.

With the proceeds of a collection made among members of the Institute to honour her memory an annual lecture was founded; the first lecture was given appropriately by Dr Fairbairn, representative of the Institute on the CMB, and again appropriately he chose as his subject 'The Importance of a Sound Training for Practising Midwives'. This was to become the main feature of the Institute's activities during the following decade.

It was suitable, therefore, that the midwife elected to the presidency of the Midwives' Institute in 1919, on the retirement of Miss Amy Hughes, was someone who had been practically concerned with the problems of training throughout the country. She was Miss A.C. Gibson, formerly president of the Birmingham Midwives' Association, and from her arrival in London chairman of the Institute's Representatives Committee. This was a committee which met at Buckingham Street on the third Friday of each month to discuss the affairs of the affiliated associations up and down the country. Miss Gibson had personally concerned herself with the formation and organisation of local associations, and thus was authoritatively placed to enlarge the Institute's sphere of influence.

It had long been ironic that the midwives had their Institute and their Act, and thus had a sound base for public recognition, while the nurses did not.

During and after the First World War that was rectified. The College of Nursing was set up in March 1916 and a Nurses' Act became law in December 1919, creating the General Nursing Council.

As so often, social and administrative reform is planned during a war and implemented as soon as possible afterwards. One of the first steps towards the creation of that 'land fit for heroes' so ambitiously planned (and perhaps so poorly executed) was the creation in 1919 of a Ministry of Health, as a means of coordinating the country's public health services. The first Secretary was fortunately a man of vision and enterprise, and Sir Robert Morant recognised that the training and provision of midwives was becoming an urgent necessity.

In 1921 the midwives' representation on the Central Midwives' Board was strengthened when the Institute was invited to nominate two members, both practising midwives. They were both members of Council – Miss Elizabeth Pearson (for long organiser of the affiliated associations) and Miss Pollard, Inspector of Midwives for Middlesex and the first non-medical superintendent of Midwives. The Ministry of Health appointed as its representative Miss Olive Haydon, an approved teacher, superintendent of a training school for midwives and also a member of Council. Joining the redoubtable Miss Paget, who was now celebrating her twentieth year as a member of CMB, they ensured that the Institute and its midwives had a strong voice in the Board's deliberations.

But it was the education of midwives that preoccupied the Institute during the twenties, and the co-ordinating of their activities. As Miss Pearson said in the Fynes-Clinton Lecture of 1922:

'We have about 70 associations, branching out from this Institute like fingers from a hand . . . But this is not enough. There are still vast spaces in the country untouched by us . . . There comes a time in all healthy concerns when the off-shoots grow beyond the detailed management of the parent body. It is a trying time, but it has to be faced, and I believe that the time has come for us to adjust our relationship with outlying districts.

One reason for the isolation of midwives in those years was the fact that the great majority of mothers had their babies at home; in 1930 hospital confinements were only 24 per cent. Not least because so many midwives were going out into a life of independent practice, when the standard of their work would be ruled by their own personal professionalism, apart from those sometimes bureaucratic local supervising authorities. Training, then, was crucial; and in 1926 several projects came to fruition to improve the standards of midwifery training. After several years' gestation, the Institute devised its own advanced course of instruction for teachers, culminating in a voluntary examination leading to the award of a diploma. In the first year, out of twenty-seven entrants six were successful (the examination was transferred to the CMB in 1930). In that year, too, the courses in midwifery provided by an increasing number of maternity hospitals were lengthened from four months to one year. And because more trained nurses were turning to midwifery to supply the admitted shortage, the period of midwifery training for the SRN and RSCN was reduced from one year to six months.

Stirrings of trade unionism were also to be strongly heard at this time, when the Bermondsey Borough Council issued a diktat that its midwives must belong to a trade union. With an acerbity that was to become familiar in later years *Nursing Notes* commented that 'nursing and midwifery are not *trades* but *professions*'; and eventually Bermondsey was persuaded to accept that 'membership of a professional association, society or institute should be deemed to be compliance with the Council's resolution'.

The great names of the early days of the Midwives' Institute were now departing. Amy Hughes, staunch president during the First World War, died in 1923. Emma Brierly, who had (at times single-handed) edited and managed *Nursing Notes* as an articulate and influential voice for the profession, died in 1924 (Rosalind Paget's niece and nephew, Miss Kathleen and Major Guy Paget, formed a limited company to continue the journal); and Jane Wilson (Mrs Brian Wilson), president during the critical Edwardian period, died in 1925.

If the loss of these great figures was saddening, that sadness was compounded in 1926 by the death in office of the incumbent president, Miss Anne Campbell Gibson, whose great and varied experience had been invaluable. She had worked in the Poor Law Service, particularly at the Brownlow Hill Workhouse hospital in Liverpool. Then she had been for twenty-four years Matron of the Birmingham Poor Law Infirmary, and a leading figure in the association of midwives in that city. She had been a Nightingale nurse, trained at St Thomas's (and it had been Florence Nightingale herself who had directed her interests towards poor law nursing).

She was succeeded by another Nightingale nurse – Miss Lucy Ramsden, who had spent most of her life, latterly as Matron, at the Rotunda Lying-in Hospital in Dublin, a leading centre for midwifery training. Unfortunately Miss Ramsden was not well, and her term of office was ended by her death in the autumn of 1928.

This was a challenging time for the midwives. At last the problems of childbirth were becoming a matter for public discussion, and the provision of midwives a matter of national concern. In 1928 a group of women who had interested themselves in these matters from a voluntary standpoint set up the National Birthday Trust Fund. They were led by Lady Cholmondley, aided by Lady Rhys Williams and Mrs Stanley Baldwin. Mrs Baldwin's personal and detailed interest in the work was profoundly important, since she was the wife of the Prime Minister.

In 1928 the Ministry of Health set up a Departmental Committee to enquire into the training and practice of midwives and their conditions of employment. In 1929, another committee was set up to examine the causes of a maternal mortality that was still about 4 per 1,000 births, a figure that had not changed for some years and seemed to resist all efforts to reduce it. The Midwives' Institute welcomed both investigations and provided evidence for them; and welcomed also the conclusions of the first Departmental Committee that there should be an expansion of the midwife's training and that a national maternity and midwifery service should be set up. This proposal was strengthened by the report of the Departmental Committee on Maternal Deaths that demonstrated that there had been a 'primary avoidance factor' in 40 per cent of such deaths, generally an infection introduced by those attending the mother.

These findings supported the arguments so long put forward by the Midwives' Institute, and ensured that it had a vital part to play in the reforms that followed. Providentially, the midwives elected to be their president from January 1929 a woman whose strength, energy and unshakable determination was to be vital in the years that followed. She was Miss Edith Pye, a member of the Institute for twenty-three years, a Quaker, who had been made a Chevalier of the Legion d'Honneur for her work at a front-line maternity hospital at Chalons-sur-Marne during the war for the Friends Relief Organisation.

The importance now allotted to midwifery by the medical profession was reflected by the foundation in 1929 of the (Royal) College of Obstetricians and Gynaecologists. One of its founders (and second president) was Dr J. S. Fairbairn, formerly the Midwives' Institute representative on the CMB; another was the eighty-one-year-old Sir Francis Champneys. Sir Francis died in 1930, having been chairman of the Central Midwives' Board from its inception twenty-eight years before. He had been a staunch friend to the midwife, and in his long and dedicated service had observed, and contributed powerfully to, the transition from an antiquated and dangerously unlearned midwifery practice to a modern, well-trained and proud profession.

The Times said of him that 'his chief claim to remembrance lies in the tact and ability with which he guided a remarkable reform in the education of midwives in this country'. Sometimes his thoughtfulness was misconstrued. In the early examinations of practising midwives he realised that the unlettered ladies would not understand Latin medical terms, so he directed the examining doctors to use Anglo-Saxon English terms instead. One of the midwives came out of the examining room much offended. She said: 'The gentlemen were so *coarse*!'

Another loss that year was Marion Olive Haydon ('Sister Olive'), who died in October 1930. She had trained under Dr Annie McCall, that early supporter of the Midwives' Institute, at Clapham Maternity Hospital, and obtained her London Obstetrical Society diploma in 1901. She succeeded the legendary Mrs Messenger as head midwife and teacher of midwives at the General Lying-in Hospital, and it was as a teacher that she became invaluable to the Institute for she was the first organiser and director of the teachers' instruction course and examiner at the first teachers' examination held there. As a member of the Institute Council from 1914, a vice president from 1928, and also a member of the CMB (on the nomination o the Ministry of Health), it was appropriate that the Institute founded lecture series in her memory.

The Jubilee of the Midwives Institute was celebrated in 1931. A series o meetings took place during the first weekend in July. A jubilee fund hac been inaugurated, and on the Friday at Buckingham Street a quarterl meeting of council and a monthly meeting of the Committee of Branche and Affiliated Associations were held concurrently, at which Mrs Baldwin presented a cheque to the jubilee fund on behalf of the National Birthda' Trust. At this meeting also, the president Miss E.M. Pye presented Mis Rosalind Paget (now seventy-five, but as vigorous and incisive as ever) witl a silver medallion with the figure of an angel watching over a mother and baby, with the words: 'as a token of love from the members of Council'.

On Saturday 4 July the jubilee fund was presented at a meeting a Bedford College attended by 300 midwives from many parts of the country A message was read from the Queen:

'I have heard with interest of the celebrations in connection with the Jubile of the Midwives Institute. I congratulate the members on their fine recor of achievement, which owes much to the life-long devotion of the senio member, under whose inspiration I trust this noble cause will meet witl increasing prosperity.

The great value to the Community of the daily work of midwives i inestimable.'

MARY R.

The sum collected for the jubilee fund was then handed over to th indefatigable honorary treasurer (Rosalind Paget), together with a bool recording the names of the donors. Miss Paget responded with an amusin speech about the pioneers and founders; honoured by the Queen's messag as 'senior member', she was better qualified than anyone to look back witl pride.

As the assembled midwives at a special commemorative service in S Paul's Cathedral on Sunday 5 July sang the hymn 'Through the night o doubt and sorrow' they could be thankful for fifty years of work well done in the face of ignorance and obstruction,

Chasing far the gloom and terror,
Brightening all the path we tread.

THREE

From Belgrave Street to Mansfield Street

In the spring of 1933 the National Birthday Trust Fund came forward with a proposal that the Fund, the Queen's Institute for District Nursing and the Midwives' Institute should be housed together, and at virtually no cost to the Institute. This resolved what had become an increasing problem. The rooms at Buckingham Street were wholly inadequate for the programmes of training that the Institute now wished to introduce; moreover, the office space was uncomfortably cramped. For the past few years there had been worries that Buckingham Street itself would be swept away to build a new Charing Cross bridge. The industrial recession and mass unemployment made that less likely, but the future accommodation for the Institute was insecure.

The offer from the National Birthday Trust came at the right time. A house (given by its chairman, Sir Julian Cahn) had been found in Lower Belgrave Street, on the corner of Eaton Square, near Victoria. The Midwives' Institute would have office accommodation, a members' club-room on the third floor, and five bedrooms for the use of members visiting London. It was a generous offer and the Institute accepted it.

The new building was opened in October, and Queen Mary visited it within a week of its opening. It was a working day, and the Queen was interested to listen to the Council of the Institute in session. She was also taken to see the members' room, and her sharp eye noticed that it had no clock. On the next day a handsome electric clock was delivered as a present from the Queen: No. 57 Lower Belgrave Street was now properly equipped.

Six months later there was another gesture of Royal favour when the International Midwives Union held its sixth Annual Congress in London. Miss Pye, as president of the host nation's midwives' organisation, took the chair for a great series of meetings of 305 members; ten countries sent delegates, and five others were represented by individuals, including India and China. On the evening before the Congress formally opened the delegates were received by the Patron of the Congress, Her Royal Highness the Duchess of York*, herself a mother – her daughter, the Princess Elizabeth, having been born two years earlier. The *Midwives' Chronicle* commented: 'we feel proud and happy to think we have a Royal mother so distinguished for her interest in the humblest mothers of the country, to welcome our guests from overseas'. The then Duchess of York thus began fifty years of personal interest in, and concern for, the work of British midwives.

* *Now HM Queen Elizabeth the Queen Mother.*

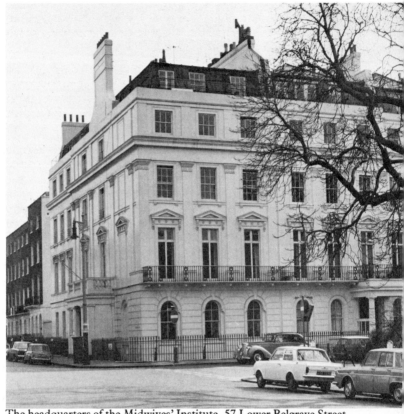

The headquarters of the Midwives' Institute, 57 Lower Belgrave Street

It was a fitting mark of the new dignity now being achieved, largely through the efforts of the Midwives' Institute, that in the autumn of 1934 the CMB revised its rules in one small but significant particular. Hitherto the midwife had been entitled to call herself 'certified midwife' adding, if appropriate, 'by examination'. But she was not allowed to abbreviate that designation. From 1934 the midwife was permitted to call herself 'State Certified Midwife' and to put after her name the initials 'S.C.M.'

The early thirties were difficult years for midwives, as they were for the country. The economic recession, leading to mass unemployment, was accompanied by a falling birthrate and there was a surplus of midwives. However, the slump meant that many plans for improvements in the national life had to be shelved, among them those for a national maternity service. Local authorities were also short of money, and not many of them were exercising their authority to pay the fees of domiciliary midwives 'in necessitous cases'. Of 61 County Councils, only 16 were paying; of 83 County Borough Councils, only 43 were paying; and of 289 other District and Borough Councils, only 46 were paying.

The rate of maternal mortality remained at the level of four in every thousand births, and was indeed rising. The first report of the Departmental Committee on Maternal Mortality in 1932 said that

'there is too little ante-natal supervision by general practitioners and midwives, and what there is often too perfunctory to deserve the name. Antenatal clinics are too often conducted by those who are not practised obstetricians, and there is a lack of coordination between them and those conducting the deliveries.'

The trend, encouraged by the medical profession, was towards hospital confinement, and in 1932 one-sixth of all births in Britain were in hospital (there had been a notable expansion of hospital maternity provision, particularly in London).

In its efforts to bring down the maternal mortality rate the Institute was strengthened by a new professionalism, and by the association with the eminent members of the National Birthday Trust. In January 1934 the Trust set up a Joint Committee on Midwifery, under the chairmanship of the Earl of Athlone (the brother of Queen Mary). There were three Institute members on that Committee, led by Miss Pye, the president. Also on the Committee was Mrs Stanley Baldwin, wife of the Prime Minister.

The Silver Jubilee of the reign of King George V was celebrated in the summer of 1935, and the Midwives' Institute had particular reason to be pleased with the Birthday Honours, for Rosalind Paget – who after nearly forty years' dedicated service as their honorary treasurer had just given up the office – was appointed a Dame of the Most Noble Order of the British Empire. Though now an old lady, she was still straight-backed and intensely interested in the doings of 'her midwives'; and one of the special celebrations she most enjoyed was a teaparty held to honour her at Lower Belgrave Street, organised by the secretary, Miss Simpson.

The Joint Committee on Midwifery duly reported in 1935 and proposed the creation of a salaried midwifery service. This received powerful backing from the London County Council which passed a resolution supporting the recommendation 'subject to a satisfactory grant-in-aid from national funds, but . . . the Council was not in agreement with the proposals to pay compensation to certain classes of practising midwives and to give pensions in certain circumstances'.

The Midwives' Institute had introduced its own contributory pension scheme for midwives in 1929, but this was not designed to recompense women who, not wishing to join a national scheme, might have their means of livelihood thus arbitrarily taken away. In principle the Institute was in favour of a salaried scheme, but insisted on the rights of the independent midwife being upheld, and adequate compensation being provided for those who might be harmed by the introduction of a scheme wholly under the control of the local authorities.

Miss Pye said that 'in rural areas where there have been salaried midwives under County Nursing Associations for many years, there is no freedom of choice for the mother, but where an efficient midwife is provided, and there is the added safeguard of the right type of supervision, this is not a cause of complaint'. The Institute put in its own memorandum that practising midwives should have an opportunity to join the service, but that those who were not accepted should be generously compensated. 'Every effort should be made to preserve a personal relationship between mother and midwife'. The Institute noted that there was no intention to prevent the practice of the independent midwife. During the period of transition, as much as possible should be done to encourage their cooperation with the public services.

King George V died in January 1936; the Institute sent a message of condolence to Queen Mary. The new King, Edward VIII, was a bachelor and evidently it was not thought fitting for the midwives to communicate with him. Indeed, it is interesting that practically no mention of him was made in *Nursing Notes*; when the following December he abdicated, it was once again to his mother, Queen Mary, that the Institute sent a message of sympathy.

That year has gone down in history as the year of the Abdication. Much has been made of the fact (he mentioned it in his Abdication broadcast) that the future Duke of Windsor did not enjoy a stable family life with wife and children, such as that so valued by his brother the Duke of York, who now became King George VI. It was ironic that in the year of a troubled bachelor king a major stride forward should have been made in midwifery provision.

Not least of the reasons for this was the positive support of the Prime Minister. Stanley Baldwin said in the House of Commons in January 1936 that 'there was a subject which had been near his heart for many years before he had attained a position where he might have a hand in putting it through. This was the question of maternity and midwives. Here was a question upon which there could be no political conflict. He would try to peg out a claim now early by begging the House to see when they came to that Bill that if it commended itself to the House they might do their best to get it through this session'.

The Institute held a series of meetings with representatives from all parts of the country. At this time there were some 60,000 midwives on the Roll of the Central Midwives Board (though only about 10 per cent of them were paid-up members of the Institute). It was estimated that about 15,000 practised. Some 8,000 worked as midwives in hospitals or nursing homes, or as salaried midwives under either the Queen's Institute of District Nursing or under county nursing associations. No more than 7,000 were in independent practice.

In the spring the Institute paused from campaigning to give a dinner to Dr John Shields Fairbairn on his retirement as chairman of the CMB (he had succeeded Sir Francis Champneys, and for twelve years before had been the Midwives' Institute representative on the Board).

He had been a keen advocate of training for midwives, and at the General Lying-in Hospital he was the moving spirit in the establishment at Camberwell of the first post-certificate school for midwives. He was one of the first examiners for the midwives' Teachers' Diploma (and author of a standard text-book). He insisted that the Institute should be the best teaching centre in London, and took charge of the 'Fairbairn and Paget Lecture Course'. As a founder of the Royal College of Obstetricians and Gynaecologists, he was well placed to improve the historically uneasy relationship between the midwives and some members of the medical profession, and that he largely achieved. Personally a friendly and sympathetic man, he was proud to be given a special present by his midwife friends: a chair which, in the eight years of his retirement at Lossiemouth, he made his own, always referring to it as 'the midwives' chair'.

The third Midwives' Act came into operation on 31 July 1936. It was intended

'to secure the organisation throughout the country of a domiciliary service of salaried midwives under the control of local supervising authorities as an important step in the improvement of the maternity services and in the campaign for reducing maternal mortality. At the same time, the whole status of the midwifery profession will be raised by providing adequate salaries and secure prospects for those midwives who enter the new service, and by compensating those who retire within a specified period and so reducing the present overcrowding in the ranks of the profession.'

It was laid down that local supervising authorities might employ salaried midwives themselves, or arrange for their employment by maternity and child welfare authorities, or by welfare organisations. In setting up those arrangements, the authorities must consult voluntary organisations, general practitioners, 'and local organisations of midwives (if any)'.

Local organisations of midwives were thus given a special status, and this led to a resurgence of interest in the Institute by midwives up and down the country. This interest coalesced in a great meeting held at Central Hall, Westminster, on 11 November 1936, called by the Midwives' Institute and attended by 1,200 members from 107 branches. Described at the time as 'incomparably the most important meeting that the Institute has ever held', it was addressed by the Minister of Health, Sir Kingsley Wood. He showed himself to be a good and informed friend of the midwife.

'There is nothing in these proposals that casts reflection upon the work of the independent midwives of this country (he said) . . . The position of a midwife is at least as important as that of a Health Visitor. I have suggested to the local authorities that they should adopt scales of salary which are comparable with those applicable to Health Visitors employed in the same district. The Act . . . empowers the Central Midwives Board to include in their rules a requirement that midwives should from time to time attend a course of instruction approved by the Board . . . Every local supervising authority is required to provide or arrange for the provision of courses of instruction.'

Mrs Stanley Baldwin was at this meeting. So was Dame Rosalind Paget, who may well have reflected that this was a greater tribute to her achievement over half a century: the contrast between those few women meeting together in Buckingham Street, and this mass of well over a thousand midwives meeting the Minister of Health, must certainly have warmed her heart. This meeting was the first to be arranged by the Institute's newly-elected general and organising secretary, Mrs F.R. Mitchell.

Mrs Mitchell had been a member of the Institute from 1916, and deputy chairman of Council (she had been chairman of the Public Health and Maternity and Child Welfare Committee of a local authority). The Institute had elected her as their representative to the CMB in the previous February, but she chose to resign on becoming general secretary, to avoid any conflict of interest. Her professionalism and drive, together with her experience in local government, were to prove invaluable.

Forty-two new branches of the Institute were formed in 1936, making a total of 150. The Midwives' Institute could now claim, more powerfully than ever before, to be speaking for midwives throughout the country. It could put forward salary proposals, and argued that the midwife's salary should be 'not less than £200 per annum, with other professional costs (heating, lighting, cleaning and professional laundry) of 3s. 6d. per week, and £10 uniform allowance'. It was even envisaged that 'the midwife could be connected by telephone with a central office and could notify the office by telephone when she goes out and when she returns, unless she is off duty'. The modern midwife for whom the telephone is an essential and all-too-demanding instrument may look back wistfully at the days when her predecessor could do without one.

Some older midwives did suffer hardship as a result of the new Act's provisions. The Institute set up a temporary department to help them, in particular by establishing a clearing-house to find employment for any made redundant. A 'Million Penny' fund was started to provide financial aid; and as longer term assistance for similar future contingencies, sickness and accident insurance policies were introduced.

The Constitution of the Institute was brought up to date at this time. In the original Constitution, members were those who had signed the original Articles of Association 'and such other persons as hereinafter mentioned . . .' Only one original signatory (Dame Rosalind) remained; and so the main qualification for membership became that of State Certified Midwife, or holder of the Certificate of the Central Midwives Board 'or of any other body authorised by Parliament'; there would also be Associate and Lay Associate members, but without a vote.

Two other requirements were introduced by the CMB in these years; the length of the lying-in period of attendance by the midwife was increased from ten days to fourteen; and it was made mandatory for all practising midwives to attend a residential course of instruction for not less than four consecutive weeks in every seven years (a Ministry of Health grant of £1 a week was to be payable). The first of these refresher courses was planned for September 1939; war prevented this innovation.

The year had started well, for Queen Elizabeth had graciously agreed to be Patron of the Midwives' Institute, 'recognising as Her Majesty does the great importance to the nation of training midwives and of promoting their education and status'. The Ministry of Health was also able to report the first fall in the maternal mortality rate, to 3.13 per thousand, the lowest ever recorded in Britain, largely due to the improved standards of midwifery and the introduction from 1935 of the sulphonamide drugs.

It was satisfactory that of the 169 local supervising authorities, all had by 1939 inaugurated domiciliary midwifery services. But the most important change was that the length of training was increased to two years, with one year for State Registered Nurses.

Nevertheless the shadow of war was darkening Britain. In the last year of the peace, increasing numbers of young Jewish women were coming to Britain from Germany, Austria and Czechoslovakia to seek a haven from persecution. As chairman of the Midwives Sub-Committee of the Nursing and Midwifery Department of the Coordinating Committee for Refugees, Miss Pye put in much devoted organisation to enable those with nursing qualifications to complete their midwifery training in this country.

War was declared in September 1939 and for a few months the Midwives' Institute found itself homeless (though the reason for leaving Lower Belgrave Street was a legal complication over shared responsibility for war damage, rather than any fear of bombing). For a time, the Institute operated from the home of the general secretary, Mrs Mitchell, at 20 Selwood Road, Croydon. However, in January 1940 the offices reopened once more in central London.

In that month also the particular nature of the midwives' house journal was recognised by a change of title: *Nursing Notes and Midwives' Chronicle* became, as it had long been, the *Midwives' Chronicle and Nursing Notes*.

The main characteristic of the first year of the war was the disruption of civilian life – not least by the evacuation of expectant mothers, for whom emergency maternity homes were set up. Many thousands of children were also evacuated from the cities, an enterprise in which many rural midwives found themselves helping as surrogate mothers to resettle the children in their strange surroundings. The country prepared itself for bombing or invasion, and the Institute campaigned for the issue of steel helmets and respirators for midwives. The Ministry, as ministries will, issued ponderous directives, one laying down that in the event of a 'sudden birth in an air raid shelter', the mother 'should be regarded as an urgent casualty'.

It was in the early winter of 1941 that bombing began to bring the midwives of Britain into tough wartime conditions. One supervisor reported an incident that could have been paralleled in many cities: this happened in January 1941 –

'One midwife during a very bad air raid when a great many homes were demolished, and a good many people were killed in the village in which she works, was attending a patient in labour. She was alone in the house with the mother who fainted when the bombs were falling, and although nurse tried to get some assistance, she was unable to do so. She delivered the baby which was a breech, and attended to the mother, who recovered consciousness. When the planes passed over a neighbour helped the nurse lift a heavy deal table on to the bed to act as some protection for the mother, and the placenta was expelled. Both mother and baby made an excellent recovery. It must have been a bit nerve wracking for the midwife.'

It must indeed. The civilian services did their best to help midwives as a priority, and one midwife gave an account of running through the blitz to a case, escorted fore and aft by two policemen, and on either side of her, two air raid wardens.

Their work was acknowledged in a letter to *The Times* from the president of the Royal College of Obstetricians and Gynaecologists, W. Fletcher Shaw:

'To a woman in this time of supreme strain the presence of a highly trained, sympathetic midwife means much: how much more in the dangers and horrors of an aerial bombardment, only those who have endured it can tell. The work of these midwives is known, however, to those who receive their reports, the supervisors of midwives and the doctors, who not infrequently share their dangers and anxieties, and it is they who have asked me to voice their appreciation of the gallant way the midwives have carried out their duties and to remind the nation of the debt of gratitude it owes to them.'

The year 1941 marked the diamond jubilee of the Midwives' Institute. Though it was no time for lavish celebration, there was a modest ceremony in Tuke Hall, Bedford College at which the National Birthday Trust presented a cheque to begin the 'Jubilee Fund', with which it was hoped in better times to provide the Institute with a home of its own. A badge was designed for the use of members, representing the tree of life with its roots in the year of foundation (1881) and spreading out into its branches, representing each and every one of its members. On the badge was inscribed the motto 'Vita Donum Dei' – 'Life is the Gift of God'.

It was in 1941 that Mrs Florence Mitchell completed twenty-five years' work for the College, and was presented with a cheque. The Council also decided that she should have an assistant, and Miss Marjorie Bayes was appointed to this new post.

The importance of the Institute in promoting and carrying out the training of midwives was now generally acknowledged; and it was felt that this body was no longer simply an 'Institute', but could rightly and properly call itself a 'College', a home and centre of education. So after due enquiries – the Queen approved the change, and the Board of Trade was prepared to sanction it – an extraordinary general meeting was held in December 1941 at which the College of Midwives was created out of the Midwives' Institute. The modest luncheon at the Savoy that followed this meeting became, as one speaker felicitously remarked, 'more a christening than a jubilee'.

In the following summer, at Lady Margaret Hall, Oxford, 150 midwives gathered from all parts of the country for the first one-week residential summer school on midwifery. The inaugural lecture was given by the Chairman of the Central Midwives' Board, Sir Comyns Berkeley, who took the opportunity to support the midwives in their campaign for better pay and status:

'In the future I can visualise your College taking an honoured place among the Colleges of England (he said). To attain such an object, however, you must do all in your power to advance the status of your College, take pride in it and love it . . .

I feel that the time is coming, and must come, when the profession of midwives will attain a position both in the public estimation and in that of other collegiate bodies which is its right . . . The profession of midwives is among the most important in the country . . .'

It was true that there was a shortage of midwives; although more were being trained, and well trained, many were choosing not to practice because the pay and conditions were so inadequate. This was implicitly acknowledged by the setting up of an official Midwives Salaries Committee under the chairmanship of Lord Rushcliffe.

That the midwives were now a well-educated and intellectually aware group is demonstrated by the appearance in the pages of the *Midwives' Chronicle* of articles about new medical advances. In December 1942 John Hatcher wrote an article on 'penicillin, a new bacteriostatic'. 'Knowledge is still in its infancy', he wrote, 'however, many competent authorities consider the discovery may well prove to be one of the outstanding medical discoveries of this war'.

Despite the challenges and difficulties of the war years the extension of training was carried forward by the College. The one-week residential course at Oxford in 1942 was a notable success and was repeated in the following year. In 1944 the demand was so great that two courses had to be held. Meanwhile, with the encouragement of the College, a number of local branches began to organise intensive refresher courses in their neighbourhoods. To coordinate this movement, Miss Mary Hurry was appointed the College's first education officer in 1944 (she died, at the tragically young age of thirty-seven, three years later). Soon postgraduate schools lasting for one week had been held in Bangor, Bristol and London. Meanwhile the College itself had been approved as a lecture centre for Part II pupil lectures. A scholarship was established by the Council named after Mr Arnold Walker, in gratitude for his work as chairman of the Midwives Panel of the Midwives Salaries Committee. In addition a research scholarship was founded to enable a midwife to assist a doctor who was undertaking research into the use of analgesia in childbirth.

During the war many people in government and in the professional bodies were looking forward to the peace, and laying plans for the brave new world that they trusted would emerge from the years of conflict. In 1943 the 'Beveridge Report' was published, and set in train discussions on the future form of national insurance and social provision generally, including the health services. The Government's blueprint for a National Health Service was published in a White Paper in the spring of 1944; and once more it seemed that the midwives had been ignored. The College of Midwives published its comments: 'The aim of the new health service should be to keep the midwifery service by midwives as an important and independent public service . . . There is, unfortunately, no clear-cut account of the midwives' part in the service'.

At the General Election of July 1945, a Labour Government was over-whelmingly voted into office with the Rt Hon Clement Attlee as Prime Minister. He appointed Mr Aneurin Bevan as Minister of Health; and the long negotiations began for the launching of the National Health Service three years later.

It was a time for cooperation, and so it was fitting that in 1946 the Scottish Midwives Association decided to amalgamate with the College of Midwives. The autonomy of Scotland – expressed officially by the continuance of a separate and distinct Central Midwives Board for Scotland – was recognised by the creation of a separate Council in Edinburgh which was known as the College of Midwives, Scottish Council. The eight Scottish branches then existing were thus brought more closely into touch with affairs in London. That the merger was achieved so effectively and in such an amicable spirit was in no small measure due to the work of Miss Jean Ferlie, chairman of the Scottish Midwives Association at this time, and Mrs F.R. Mitchell, the general secretary of the College.

At about the same time, the Ulster Midwives Association was reorganised to form the Northern Ireland Council of the College of Midwives. This was the earnest wish of Miss Marjorie Sparkes, for long a member of the Midwives' Institute, who arranged for the Ulster Midwives Association to become affiliated to the Midwives' Institute in 1938. The president of the Northern Ireland Council was Miss Clark-Kennedy, Matron of the Royal Maternity Hospital, Belfast, with Miss Sparkes as vice-president. Thus by 1946 the College of Midwives could claim to speak for the midwives of England, Wales, Scotland and Northern Ireland.

As if to demonstrate this new unity, a state uniform for midwives was introduced that year. It consisted of a mid-grey coat with facings of madonna blue, with a madonna blue gingham indoor dress.

The College was being called upon more and more to act as a representative body. 'Much of its work, although it is not a Trades Union (wrote the president in 1947), falls within the category of that undertaken by a negotiating body. At the meetings of the Midwives Salaries Committee the members of the Midwives' Panel which represents midwives' interests, and of which 50 per cent of the members are representatives of the College of Midwives – confer with the Employers' Panel with a view to agreeing salaries and conditions of service of midwives'.

The status of the College became a material issue when in 1947 Willesden Borough Council served notices of dismissal, signed by the Medical Officer of Health, on nurses and midwives in the employ of the Council, including the matrons of the municipal hospital and the maternity hospital, and domiciliary midwives who refused to join a trade union. The nurses and midwives who had not been dismissed immediately agreed to support those dismissed, and eight midwives at the maternity hospital handed in their notice, saying that they would leave if the Council's notices were not withdrawn. The Council reconsidered, and agreed to recognise as negotiating bodies for nurses and midwives the Royal College of Nursing, the Royal British Association of Nurses and the College of Midwives. The notices were withdrawn and the doctors and nurses reinstated.

In that year the College devised another new constitution. There were to be four grades of membership: midwives, professional associates (ie. SRN with Part I certificate of the CMB or other professional qualification), lay associates, and pupil midwives. The president was to serve for three years, and be eligible for a second term of three years, but not eligible again for a further three. Finally, and perhaps most important, Council would be elected by regional voting; there would be three regions and six areas, and two members would be elected by each area, a total of thirty-six. The Annual General Meeting for 1947 was held in May at County Hall, London, and 300 midwives attended. They proceeded to break their own new rules by electing Miss Edith Pye their president for a twentieth year. Unwillingly, she accepted; but it was happy that she did, for in the next month, by command of the King, the former Midwives' Institute was granted the Royal Charter by which it became the Royal College of Midwives.

The National Health Service came into being on 5 July 1948. It introduced the principle that medical care and treatment should be free for all citizens. The change that most profoundly affected midwives was that, until 1948, mothers requiring the attendance of a doctor at childbirth had to pay his fee. Now every mother could (in theory) summon a doctor without payment. There was therefore some understandable apprehension among midwives that their professional function would be supplanted by the doctors.

The administrative division of the National Health Service which set up a 'tripartite' arrangement for the midwifery services was a further cause of worry. All maternity hospitals and homes were transferred from the local health authorities to regional hospital boards, while the local health authorities continued to administer the domiciliary midwives, and executive councils controlled the general practitioners and thus the maternity medical services. The RCM (as we shall now refer to the Royal College of Midwives) was disturbed that this arrangement perpetuated the division between hospital work and domiciliary midwifery: there was a danger of lack of coordination between the hospitals and the home. It was felt that this might be solved where the local health authority gave responsibility for the domiciliary service to the maternity hospital.

The midwives' fears that they would become subordinate to the overriding control of the doctors proved to be largely groundless, not least because of the pressure of demand on the doctors. Gradually, and over a period of some years, the division of responsibilities was agreed; and while the majority of women did ask for both a doctor and a midwife, in 75 per cent of cases the midwife conducted the delivery. In fact, a more substantial change in the responsibilities of domiciliary midwives came from the trend towards hospital confinement, which brought about the situation that domiciliary midwifery was to be involved with ante-natal and post-natal care for mothers and babies while the actual birth, which the midwives were trained and qualified to assist, took place in hospital.

If the place of midwives in the National Health Service took some time to settle down, at least the midwives were recognised as professionals with an indispensable function to perform. It was a tribute to the 'Florence Nightingale of midwifery', Dame Rosalind Paget, who died on 19 August 1948 at her niece's home in Sussex at the age of ninety-three. That the RCM exists is in great part due to her; its story is her story. A trust fund was set up to commemorate her, as she would certainly have wished, by providing travelling scholarships for midwives; and, as a further commemoration, the members of the RCM subscribed to a fund which provided bookshelves for the library (now in the members' room).

Another great figure died that year – Miss A.A.I. Pollard, one of the first Superintendents of Midwives. Her tall, commanding figure, and her articulate and incisive contributions to committee meetings and to the Central Midwives Board, were greatly missed. Miss Edith Simpson died in 1949; she had preceded Mrs Mitchell as secretary (at Buckingham Street, from 1921) and later had acted as club secretary and librarian.

The shortage of practising midwives continued. In 1948, to improve this situation the RCM organised two four-month courses for midwife teachers, and the Government provided scholarships to encourage qualified midwives to take these courses. Nevertheless when the Health Ministry's Maternity Liaison Committee, which became the Working Party on Midwives (chaired by Mrs Mary Stocks, then principal of Westfield College, London) reported in 1949 it referred to the problem of an 'absolute shortage' of midwives.

The Working Party recommended that Maternity Services Committees should be set up in each hospital region, to include obstetricians, general practitioners and midwives. Every local health authority should appoint an SCM as supervisor of midwives, and she should not be subordinate to the superintendent nursing officer. There would be no economy, the Working Party said, in integrating the midwifery services with the nursing profession. Domiciliary midwives should be helped by allowances for domestic help, and for running cars. Finally, the authority of the RCM was confirmed by a recommendation that the election of midwife representatives on the CMB should be through the Royal College, and not by vote throughout the profession – for the practical reason that in such an arrangement, the midwives could hardly know who they were voting for, and would be simply voting for an unknown name.

The midwives' point of view was put forcefully to the Minister of Health when Mr Aneurin Bevan attended a branch meeting: 400 midwives at County Hall told him in no uncertain terms that in some areas, midwives were being relegated to the status of 'midwifery nurse'.

In fact, Aneurin Bevan took a personal interest in the midwives. They had welcomed his appointment in 1945; the *Midwives' Chronicle* wrote that 'he has become well known in the House of Commons for his fearless criticism and caustic comment – qualities which should prove of inestimable value in his new office'. That trust was not misplaced. Despite the multifarious problems of preparing and launching the National Health Service, Bevan made sure that the cause of the midwives was sustained (at just the time he was being lectured by a hall full of angry midwives, he was setting up the Midwifery and Maternity Advisory Committee). It was also in part due to his personal authority that the Midwife Teachers Training College was set up at Kingston with Miss Lois Beaulah as principal, and a plaque at the College commemorates his part in its foundation.

Having seen the RCM safely through its first year of life within the Health Service, Miss Edith Pye resigned the presidency in June 1949. She had been a member for over forty years, having joined the Midwives' Institute in 1906; and she had occupied the taxing and crucial post of president for twenty most difficult and challenging years, through the planning of the third Midwives' Act in 1936, the Second World War, and then the introduction of the National Health Service. She was a woman of extraordinary energy and concentration. In the First World War she had run a maternity hospital in France (and been awarded the Legion d'Honneur) for the Friends Relief organisation. For many years she remained on the committee of management of that hospital. In 1919, with her devoted friend Dr Hilda Clark, she went to Vienna with a Society of Friends relief unit to organise the distribution of food to mothers and children.

During the Spanish civil war she was there helping refugee children. She played a large part in providing help for refugees from Hitler's Europe. In 1940, almost inevitably, she was in France when it collapsed, as vice-chairman of the Quaker committee for refugees; for many years she was honorary secretary of the Famine Relief Committee. She had been an innovator; she had originated the chloroform capsules that were an early aid to analgesia in childbirth. But it was her meticulously disciplined mind that her friends remembered. One noticed that she was apparently able to conduct two separate conversations simultaneously – one with a visitor and the other on the telephone – and maintain the thread of each independently and clearly. Miss Pye was awarded the OBE in 1943.

She was succeeded as president by Miss Mabel Liddiard. Miss Liddiard's general and midwifery training had been at St Thomas's Hospital. She had then gone to New Zealand and trained in the method of Dr Truby King; returning to England, she had become Matron and then nursing director of the Mothercraft Training Society (from which she retired in 1945). She was the author of books on mothercraft, and an authority on breast feeding and infant care. For some years she had been chairman of the RCM Benevolent Fund committee, and chairman also of the public health sectional committee of the National Council of Women. Her gentle, soft-spoken manner endeared her. She was ably supported by Miss Kathleen Coni, Matron of the Hull Maternity Hospital who, through years in which fund-raising was to be of great importance, ably filled the role of honorary treasurer. Miss Liddiard was to be the first president to wear a chain of office, which was provided by the subscriptions of branches in 1951.

Continuity was provided at this time by Mrs F.R. Mitchell, the general secretary. If Miss Pye was a notable leader in her years as president, Mrs Mitchell was the willing workhorse. From her appointment as general secretary in 1936 to her retirement in 1952 she threw herself wholeheartedly into the work of the RCM. She travelled round the country ensuring that the branches felt themselves to be truly a part of the central organisation (and was instrumental in associating the midwives of Scotland and Northern Ireland with those of England and Wales). She dedicated her whole life and energies to the cause of the midwives; she would brook no opposition and was quite relentless in arguing their case, in any and every forum. It was a Ministry of Health senior official who said of her, only half-jokingly, 'Ah, Mrs. Mitchell! I dare not mention the word "nurse" in front of her, without adding the word "midwife"!' Her devotion was acknowledged in 1944 by the award of the OBE.

The special interests of domiciliary midwives were recognised in 1950 by the formation of the Council of Domiciliary Midwives; 105 representatives were appointed by the branches, and 103 attended the first meeting. Their particular training needs were acknowledged by the provision of an intensive course of training for district teaching midwives.

Training was now a most important function of the RCM, and it was fitting that Mrs Mitchell's successor as general secretary should be Miss Audrey Wood who had in the previous year become tutor to the non-resident midwife teachers' course. Miss Wood was the first graduate to be general secretary, which epitomised the new level of qualification being achieved by midwives; she came from Northern Ireland and had been instrumental in helping to organise the Northern Ireland Council, which gave her a particular sympathy with the provincial branches.

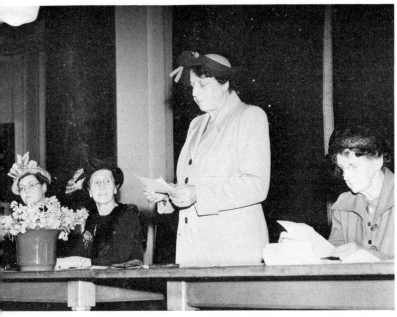

Left to right, Miss Nora Deane, Miss Mabel Liddiard, Mrs Florence Mitchell and Miss Edith Pye. *Photograph courtesy of* Nursing Mirror

It was the growing reputation of the RCM as a training centre that led to its increasing importance internationally. If Britain was declining as a world power, its lead as a powerhouse of training for the professions was if anything being enlarged. The first overseas enquiry after the Second World War came from Uruguay, as a result of which a Spanish-speaking nurse from Montevideo came to London to do her midwifery training. Shortly afterwards the New Zealand Army sent a nurse. It was not long before the trickle became a flood; the RCM was placing as many as 300 overseas students in British hospitals. Meanwhile an enquiry was received from midwives in Sweden asking whether the pre-war international congresses of midwives could not be revived; and in 1949, to coincide with the Maternity and Child Welfare Conference in London, an international meeting of midwives was held at Lower Belgrave Street, attended by representatives from eight European countries.

Five years of planning followed, much of the groundwork being laid by the assistant secretary of the RCM, Miss Marjorie Bayes. The success of her work was evident at Tuke Hall, Bedford College, London in September 1954 when 800 midwives from 46 countries heard the Minister of Health (the Rt Hon Iain McLeod) say that 'If there is one feature of our British Health Services in which we feel unrestrained pride it is our midwifery service'. As a result of this congress, in 1955 the International Confederation of Midwives was formed and its headquarters placed in London, at the

RCM, with Miss Bayes as its executive secretary.

One popular feature of the international congress was a film, 'The British Midwife', sponsored for the RCM by Cow & Gate Ltd and 'starring' a real midwife, Mrs Marjorie Gregory of Kent.

The president of the RCM at the international congress was Miss Nora Deane, who had succeeded Miss Liddiard in 1952. Miss Deane was Matron of Bristol Maternity Hospital, where she had created a tradition of high professionalism (she insisted that all her Sisters had to be midwife teachers). She had great presence and intelligence and was an excellen public speaker. Her work for the RCM was much helped by the generosity she received from her local hospital board, which wholeheartedly supported her extra-mural activities.

A Ministry of Health report on the first five years of the National Health Service, to 1953, demonstrated that the work done by midwives was changing; its scope had been increased, with the increase in ante-natal clinics, and in some areas an extension of the attendance period beyond fourteen days. The falling birthrate had produced lighter case-loads, but it was good to see 'a steady growth of cooperation with doctors'. There were 7,352 domiciliary midwives employed under the NHS, of whom 6,388 were employed by local authorities, and 964 by hospitals or voluntary organisations. As an acknowledgement of this extension of the midwife's responsibilities, the Central Midwives Board in 1955 revised the rules to add to the second period of midwifery training a study of mothercraft and nutrition. From this time, also, it was required that every midwife should attend a refresher course every five years. In this same year, the upper age limit for entry to midwifery training was raised to forty. It was becoming customary for more married women to return to work once their children had reached school age, and this provision allowed those with nursing qualifications to consider midwifery as a profession.

The chairman of the CMB, Mr Arnold Walker, said that 'compared with 20 years ago, the midwife now carries less clinical responsibility than she did, but against this, her responsibilities in the field of health education are increasing. Maternal and peri-natal mortality are steadily declining, and can be made to decline still further. Not the least is the elimination of fear and ignorance, and here the midwife can contribute so much'. Miss Deane, the president, commented that 'although we are training more than enough pupils, we are retaining in the profession insufficient to meet the needs of the service'.

The demands being made upon the RCM in other ways were also increasing. It had become significant as a representative negotiating body, through its representatives on the Nurses and Midwives Council of the Whitley Council, the official body to establish pay and conditions of employment. It was a sponsoring body for the UK Committee of the World Health Organisation. To cope with these requirements, the permanent staff of the RCM had now increased from five to fifteen, and the office space at Lower Belgrave Street was now quite inadequate. The midwives had welcomed the hospitality of the National Birthday Trust for twenty-two years, but it was now time for a professional body to have a home of its own. Most urgently, the RCM needed classrooms for its growing training programme.

In 1953 a special Appeal Committee was set up to organise fund-raising, and in 1954 a National Appeal Fund was launched with a target of £150,000. The Building and Appeal Committee chaired by Mr C.S.B. Wentworth-Stanley CBE was responsible for planning the appeal, and for negotiations on the proposed building. Her Grace the Duchess of Argyll became Patron of the appeal. A Special Appeal Committee chaired by Lady Compton was responsible for special fund-raising efforts.

The response was swift throughout the country. The Scottish Council formed their own committee and raised £16,000; Northern Ireland despite its small membership raised £1,900, and the midwifery profession through the country raised £92,000, with generous support from regional hospital boards, hospital management committees and teaching hospitals, firms, trusts and associations. The Viscountess Savernake sponsored the 'Baby-brick' scheme under which parents of newborn infants were invited to give a donation as a 'thank-you' for the birth of their baby. The contribution, with a minimum of one shilling, went towards a brick for the new college and in return the baby became a member of the Baby Brick Club and received a membership card, blue for a boy and pink for a girl, with a picture of a small child building bricks. Lady Savernake's daughter Carina became a founder member of the scheme, which was sponsored in Scotland by Lady Minto. When it closed, 40,000 babies had 'bought' bricks.

The Scottish Council was sympathetic to the idea of a home for the RCM since it had in 1955 achieved its own first home, at 37 Frederick Street, Edinburgh; the opening by the Lady Provost of Edinburgh was attended by Miss Renwick, the chairman of the Scottish Council, and Miss Deane from London, who mentioned in particular the work for midwives of Miss Jean Ferlie of Edinburgh as a member of the Whitley Council from its inception.

There were other special contributions to the building appeal. The Nuffield Foundation provided £10,000 as an acknowledgement of the RCM's activities as an educational trust. The film 'The British Midwife' had been shown throughout the cinemas of the Rank Organisation and its chairman, Mr John Davis, presented a cheque resulting from generous donations from cinemagoers. One Sunday evening Good Cause Appeal on BBC Radio was made by an 'anonymous midwife', and produced a further generous response.

Miss Kathleen Paget presented a silver cup, once the possession of her aunt Dame Rosalind Paget, for competition among the branches: it would be held annually by the branch raising the greatest amount of money in proportion to its membership. It was won in the first year by the thirty-two members of the Holland-with-Boston branch, who had between them raised £600; they subsequently won the cup outright.

By the end of 1955 it was apparent that the necessary funds would be raised. A site had been found at 15 Mansfield Street, on the corner of New

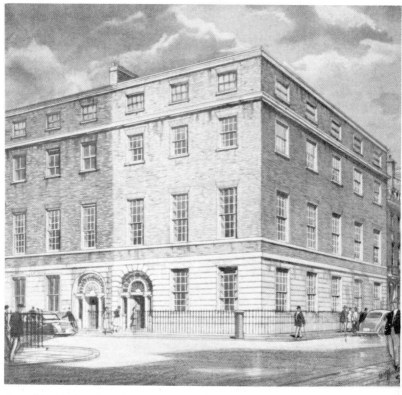

An architect's drawing of 15 Mansfield Street

Cavendish Street, between Harley Street and Portland Place, in the West End of London. An architect was appointed – Mr W.J. Biggs of Messrs E. & A. Stone, Toms & Partners – and he produced drawings of a workman-like building which would blend sensitively and undramatically with the mainly Georgian character of the remainder of the street. On 24 May 1956 the foundation stone was laid by Her Majesty Queen Elizabeth the Queen Mother, who thus renewed once again her kindness to the midwives and their institution. The Queen Mother was accompanied by Edwina, Coun-tess Mountbatten, the Duchess of Argyll and Viscountess Savernake. After the ceremony, there was a tea-party at the Royal Institute of British Architects building nearby, at which with her customary thoughtfulness the Queen Mother spoke to most of the midwives present.

Building work proceeded with admirable speed and the Royal College of Midwives was ready for occupation on 3 April 1957. As ever when a move is made to a new home, it took time to furnish, even with the generous gifts of a number of firms. The British Oxygen Company provided furnishings for the council room, Ortho-Pharmaceutical Limited for the conference room,

Boots Pure Drug Company Limited for the members' room, and John Wyeth and Brothers Limited for the President's room.

There was a further poignant reminder of Dame Rosalind Paget: her desk was appropriately placed in the library, where successive librarians might when seated at it derive a fitting sense of historical continuity. The library itself was to be named the Arnold Walker–Florence Mitchell Library, after two vice-presidents of the RCM, the former chairman of the Central Midwives Board (1946–1967) and the former general secretary.

No. 15 Mansfield Street was planned to provide administrative offices on the ground floor, a council room and smaller committee rooms, a large lecture hall seating 150, a special classroom for students preparing for the Midwives' Teachers' Diploma, the library, a members' room (with comfortable armchairs, as well as writing desks), a basement canteen, offices for the education department, and offices for the secretariat of the International Confederation of Midwives. The scale of educational work was now growing again; in addition to the postgraduate courses, midwife teachers' courses, and preliminary lecture courses, ten refresher courses were held in 1955, and sixteen (with 2,300 places) in 1956. The first course on parentcraft, group teaching and relaxation was also held that year. The successful attainment of the Mansfield Street home made it possible to continue this level of activity.

On 16 October 1957 Her Royal Highness the Duchess of Gloucester visited the RCM and unveiled a plaque to commemorate its official opening. A most happy celebration took place a month later when Miss Edith Pye, the senior past president, was driven up from her retirement home in Somerset so that she could see the RCM in its new home. She brought with her her medals, which she presented to the College. On that occasion, Miss Deane as president entertained to tea her two predecessors, Miss Pye and Miss Mabel Liddiard, and also the redoubtable former general secretary, Mrs Florence Mitchell.

It was satisfying for Miss Deane on handing over the presidency in June 1958 to Miss Mary Williams, matron of Queen Charlotte's Hospital, to be able to report that the appeal target of £150,000 had been exceeded by £2,695 4s. 6d. and that the midwives had therefore not only provided their college with a fine home of its own, but one unencumbered by any debt. Tributes were paid to the exertions of the appeal secretary, Miss Hutchinson. They were no less deserved by Miss Nora Deane, who in her distinguished six years of office had purposefully seen the scheme through from planning to fruition.

The final touch was added to the building in October 1958 when a particularly fine portrait of HM Queen Elizabeth the Queen Mother by Mr Bernard Dunston was presented to the College by Mr Ernest Taylor, chairman of Cow & Gate Limited, on behalf of that company.

The Royal College of Midwives was now properly housed and equipped for the years ahead. Behind the blue door in Mansfield Street work could proceed to plan for the future.

FOUR

Time of Challenge, Time of Change

The next years were to see the balance of midwifery care move from the home to the hospital. The number of hospital confinements had increased from 39.3 per cent in 1938 to 63.97 per cent in 1959, and the trend was continuing. It could be claimed that the standard of care had greatly improved in twenty years, with the introduction of the sulphonamides, blood transfusion, 'flying squad' services, and the antibiotic drugs. However, the pressures of this change on the hospitals led to occasional difficulties, when the hospital midwives could be overworked. The domestic midwives sometimes felt themselves being pushed out; the mothers whom they had prepared in the ante-natal phase were then taken out of their care when they went into hospital for the birth. Many at the RCM felt that this was a denial of that continuity of care, that reassurance of a familiar face and hand and voice, which was the essence of the relationship between the midwife and the mother.

The nature of care was also changing. Greater emphasis was being placed on the psychology of childbirth. In 1960, recognising this, the RCM organised a conference on Human Relationships in the Care of Mother and Baby. It was attended not only by midwives, but by physiotherapists, almoners, health visitors, doctors, paediatricians and members of the Natural Childbirth Trust.

Two more special gifts had been presented to the RCM in the closing months of 1959. Following a Council meeting on 19 October the chairman of the Scottish Council, Miss J.H. Beckett, presented a statuette of a mother and child on behalf of that Council. This most beautiful piece, copies from an original by Denis Peploe that had been erected in Lanarkshire in memory of the Scottish obstetrician William Smellie, was placed in a niche in the front hall of Mansfield Street. In the following month, a case of Dame Rosalind Paget's medals and honours was given to the RCM by her niece Lady Richmond. The medals had been in the possession of another niece, Miss Kathleen Paget, who had maintained her aunt's interest in the midwives up to her death the previous summer, by her direction of the *Midwives' Chronicle*; it had been her intention that the medals should find a home at Mansfield Street, and they were placed in the members' room.

In the summer of 1960 Miss Mary Williams (who had found the burdens of the presidency particularly onerous since she was simultaneously a working Matron) resigned and was succeeded by Miss Jean Ferlie. A stalwart of the Scottish Council, Miss Ferlie had retired the previous year as

Matron of the Simpson Memorial Maternity Pavilion in Edinburgh. Her quiet and unassuming manner hid a firm determination.

One further detail remained to define the Royal College of Midwives' status, the possession of a coat of arms. This was obtained in August 1960. If some midwives regretted the lesser importance now given to the old badge of the branching tree with its motto *Vita Donum Dei*, the new coat of arms was certainly appropriate.

The shield depicts a pair of hands, one on either side of an eight-pointed star, on an azure ground, bordered in black and white quarters (representing the day and night service by midwives). The shield is surmounted by the device used on the old badge, of a pomegranate tree encircled by an ancient crown. On either side of the shield are the supporters – on the right side Juno Lucina, goddess of women and childbearing, holding a sheaf of white lilies in one hand, and a naked child on the other arm; on the left side Hygeia, goddess of hygiene, holding in one hand a bowl, her arm entwined by a serpent. The College motto is inscribed beneath the shield.

The achievement of this coat of arms was the particular wish of Mr C.S.B. Wentworth-Stanley, who died in the previous April. On his return to England from a working lifetime in Karachi he had interested himself in hospital administration and especially the maternity services. He was a member of the management side of the Rushcliffe Midwives Salaries Committee from 1941; and when the RCM came to plan and build its own headquarters, Mr Wentworth-Stanley worked devotedly in its interest as chairman of the Building Appeal Committee.

In September 1960 the CMB amended its Rules once more. One amendment was welcomed by the RCM. The definition of 'a practising midwife' became: 'A midwife who holds herself out to attend professionally either as a midwife or a nurse upon a woman during pregnancy, labour or the lying-in period, or who so attends'. This meant that in future any midwife would always be regarded as acting as such in any maternity case, and was intended to create a mutual and inter-dependent relationship between the doctor and the midwife.

The other change was less welcome. The lying-in period was to be 'a period of not less than ten days nor more than 28', and thus the minimum period was reduced from fourteen days. This followed the recommendation of the Cranbrook Committee which had reported in 1959. That committee came to the conclusion that while there was a shortage of midwives in the hospital service, the midwifery provision within the tripartite system of maternity care was satisfactory. One cause of the pressure on hospital midwives was the introduction of a shorter working week: good in itself, this reform necessarily widened the difference between the midwife in hospital and in domestic practice.

In November 1960 the Southampton branch celebrated 50 years of existence. It was recalled that on 10 November 1910 'a meeting was held to discuss the advisability of promoting an association of midwives to be affiliated to the Midwives' Institute, Mrs Franklin [who had organised the meeting] to be Secretary *pro tem* and Mrs Harvey to assist her'. Mrs Ethel Harvey was happily able to be present at the celebratory dinner in 1960, having been honorary secretary of the branch for forty years; she died three months later, aged eighty-two.

The RCM itself celebrated its eightieth birthday in 1961. It could claim 11,000 members, and a worldwide reputation through its support for the International Confederation of Midwives. Each year the offices in Mansfield Street were hosts to nurses and midwives who came from all over the world, either to obtain the British midwifery qualification or to observe British midwifery methods. In 1959 there were nearly 400 enquiries from 49 different countries and 108 pupil-midwives were placed for training.

Some of them were present at Mansfield Street, colourful in their national dress for the occasion, when on 3 March 1961 Queen Elizabeth the Queen Mother visited the RCM to mark its eightieth birthday.

She toured the building, visiting the Education Department where a Midwife Teachers' Diploma class was in progress. Later Her Majesty wished the RCM many happy returns, cutting a large birthday cake decked with eighty candles, and then signing the visitors' book.

The RCM continued to campaign for a proper representation of midwives where decisions concerning midwifery were made. In particular, there was concern that within the Ministry of Health there was no midwifery officer, qualified and experienced in the profession, within the nursing division of the Ministry. A delegation from the RCM, supported by the Royal College of Obstetricians and Gynaecologists, was received by the Minister of Health (then the Rt Hon Enoch Powell) in November 1961. As a result of these discussions, two officers in the nursing division were given special responsibility for the midwifery services. Two years later, in 1963, a Midwifery Officer was eventually appointed; and it gave great satisfaction to the RCM that the first holder of that post was Miss Mary Williams, a past president of the College.

A popular success at this time was achieved by a film, 'To Janet – a Son' made for the RCM by Eothen Films (Medical) Ltd. Sponsored by Farleys' Infant Foods Ltd it was directed by Dr Philip Sattin at Plaistow Maternity Hospital.

Miss Frances Foxton became president of the RCM in June 1963. She was Matron of the Mothers' Hospital of the Salvation Army, and her own religious faith and ready accessibility contributed both a spiritual strength and a simple friendliness to the counsels of the College. It was not an easy time. The rising birthrate was once again putting great pressure on the midwifery services, and the demands on the hospital services stretched available resources to the point that the special requirements of the midwifery services could be overlooked. The RCM pointed out that between 70 and 80 per cent of normal deliveries both in hospital and outside were conducted by midwives with no doctor present, though the doctor might

Her Majesty the Queen Mother cuts the birthday cake at the Royal College of Midwives, 1961, watched by the president, Miss Jean Ferlie visit the mother during labour or very soon after the baby was born. In addition, the midwife was contributing far more than she had done even a decade earlier in the field of health education of the mother: she had become more of a teacher as well as a skilled practitioner. But administratively the tripartite system was showing signs of breaking down.

Two notable conferences were held in February 1964. A conference on obstetric nurse training, organised by the RCM, was attended by 150 nurses, midwives and obstetricians concerned with the three-month training proposed for the student nurse. Also in February a meeting of the Matrons and Superintendent Midwives Council was held at the Ministry of Health for serious discussions on pressing problems in the maternity services, on the theme 'Making the best use of maternity resources.'

On 8 April the first Mabel Liddiard Memorial Lecture was given by Sir Alan Moncrieff, entitled 'Breast feeding – Truby King and after' (Miss Liddiard had trained in the Truby King method, so this was a particularly appropriate subject).

In July 1964 the RCM issued a Statement of Policy on the Maternity Service.

The Maternity Service
'The College believes that the maternity service should be regarded as *one* service, although it is administered by three different authorities. If this principle is fully accepted by everybody, the barriers of the tripartite administration can be broken down, and real unity achieved.

The Midwife
It is essential that the maternity service of the future should be adequately staffed by well-trained midwives. They must be capable, at all levels, of taking their full share of responsibility, with their medical colleagues, for the care of the parturient woman and her child from early pregnancy until the end of the puerperium.

The midwife has been recognised for many years as a teacher of mothercraft, either to individuals or groups of mothers. In view of the present demand from young people for knowledge to enable them better to undertake their responsibilities as parents, greater emphasis should be given to this aspect of the midwife's training and practice.

The College welcomes the suggestion that the midwife should be in attendance for 28 days following confinement. This would give a satisfactory service to the mothers and babies, as continuity of care and guidance would be ensured, though daily visits during the latter part of this time would be unnecessary.

Place of Confinement
Until the demand for additional maternity beds is satisfied, the beds available must be used to the best advantage. Hospital confinement must be planned for those women with adverse medical, obstetric or social conditions. Those with good domestic circumstances, for whom a home confinement is considered suitable, should be encouraged to make use of the

excellent domiciliary service which is available for them. Many women prefer to be at home for their confinement, but there are some who have not had this experience and do not realise what is provided.

They should never be given the impression that if they have their baby at home they will receive a second-best service. In some parts of the country there are insufficient beds to allow all women who need hospital confinement to remain in hospital for the normal period of ten days. In those areas it is at present necessary for some mothers with suitable home conditions to go home early.

The College believes that early discharge schemes should only be regarded as a temporary emergency measure, to make it possible to provide beds *now* for all women who really need them, both for ante-natal care and delivery.

Careful planning and organisation is essential, and the women must be prepared beforehand for the possibility that they may go home early if all goes well.

If possible they should be discharged within the first 48 hours after confinement, so that continuity of care by the domiciliary midwife can be maintained. Other mothers, particularly those with bad home conditions, should remain in hospital for ten days.

The Domiciliary Service

At the present time over a quarter of a million births take place at home, that is 34 per cent of all births. In addition to this, approximately 20 per cent of mothers delivered in hospital receive most of their post-natal care at home, so that it is obvious that the domiciliary service is an absolutely essential part of the maternity service.

It must be maintained at the highest level of efficiency, the midwives being provided with the most up-to-date equipment, and car transport. There should be sufficient staff to enable them to give their undivided attention to women in labour.

Domiciliary midwives must be supported not only by general practitioner-obstetricians, with whom they work in close cooperation, but also by efficient and readily available emergency obstetric and paediatric services. The Home-Help service also needs considerable expansion to provide adequate domestic help for mothers delivered at home or discharged early from hospital. In these circumstances the domiciliary service can offer, for normal cases, a service as safe and efficient as that provided by the hospital, with the added advantage to the mother of her home surroundings.

The Hospital Service

If the maternity hospitals are to withstand the increasing pressure placed upon them, steps must be taken at once to recruit more midwives and to retain existing staff. Prospects of promotion in the midwifery profession are at present limited, and the ten-year hospital plan, by abolishing over 150 independent maternity hospitals and replacing them by maternity units of district general hospitals, will diminish rather than improve these prospects. A profession with so few first-grade administrative posts will never attract or keep leaders.

The College believes that all but the smallest units, whether or not they are training schools, should be administered by midwifery matrons, and not by the matrons of the general hospitals to which they are attached.

Midwives should be given more opportunities to take courses in administration to prepare themselves for these posts, and consideration should be given to providing a special administrative course for midwives. This should be in addition to the Midwife Teachers' Diploma, which at present is the only post-graduate midwifery qualification available.

Salaries and Conditions of Service for Midwives

If the maternity service is to be adequately staffed by midwives it is essential that the value to the community of their professional skill, and the heavy responsibilities they undertake should be fully recognised in their salary and status. The College believes that this has not yet been achieved and that salaries in both the hospital and the domiciliary field must be made more attractive.

Conditions of service, particularly with regard to arrangements for off-duty and night duty rotas, must be improved. This applies as much to the domiciliary as to the hospital service. All midwives should have sufficient clerical and auxiliary help to free them from extraneous tasks so that their knowledge and skill may be devoted to the immediate care of the mother and child, and to the teaching of the mother, the junior staff and the pupil-midwife.

Conclusion

These are challenging and exciting days and much research work is being done to evolve the best possible maternity service for the country. The Royal College of Midwives will always endeavour to be progressive in its thinking, and thereby make its full contribution towards this end.'

The introduction into hospital maternity services in 1965 of 'elective early discharge' (whereby mothers might choose to leave hospital early, thus complicating still further the relationships between the various responsibilities of the hospital and domiciliary midwives) added to the problem. It seemed that for the sake of a neat administrative hospital structure, the special skills of the midwife were to be sacrificed.

Miss Foxton, as president of the RCM, put it clearly to the congress of the Royal Society of Health in June 1965:

'The midwives of the country are dissatisfied with the present situation . . . We are not convinced that a uniform pattern of service with a single administrative head is necessarily the right answer. We are aware that various schemes are being tried out in different parts of the country and it

seems that unity of purpose is to be aimed at rather than uniform of practice
. . .'

They should try to reduce the pressure on doctors and midwives and
more especially the midwives in hospital who had recently been under fire
for not offering the mother comfort, support and insight into her personal
needs.

'How can she when the pressure of work is so great and when supporting
staff is lacking? She cannot do so as she knows she should, and this makes
for job dissatisfaction, general frustration and, eventually, capitulation –
she leaves the maternity service. The matter must be tackled at local level
since no amount of overhead legislation will provide the answer.'

A few months later, the report of a Committee on the Staffing of the
Midwifery Service in Scotland, chaired by Mrs Wolridge-Gordon, noted
that a hospital work-study had discovered that only one-third of the hospital
midwife's time was spent on work requiring her special skills; much time
was spent on administrative, clerical or domestic work.

In part, the Committee felt that this was due to the attitude of the
midwives themselves:

'Some midwives feel that they are not working unless they are doing
something with their hands; faced with the alternatives of, say, sorting out
linen, or talking to mothers, and gaining their confidence, midwives would,
it seems, feel that the first was work and the second was not. We think it
should be impressed on midwives (and pupil-midwives during their training) that teaching mothers is a very important part of their job, that this
includes not just active instruction but making opportunities for conversa-
tion with them, to give them a chance to ask advice on questions that are
troubling them'

It seems that Martha and Mary still live.

Two of the notable figures who contributed much in their different ways to
the development of the RCM died at this time: Juliet, Lady Rhys Williams
DBE, and Miss Kathleen Coni OBE. Lady Rhys Williams, a daughter of
the novelist Elinor Glyn, had followed her own career as a Hollywood
scriptwriter, and as a novelist; but returning to Wales, she conducted a
series of nutrition experiments in the Rhondda Valley, providing expectant
mothers with calories and vitamins. She was thus a pioneer of the modern
use of pre-natal foods and supplements. She also wrote books on economics,
family allowances and taxation, and was a leader of the European movement. But it was as a founder of the National Birthday Trust that she was
instrumental in providing the then Midwives' Institute with a home at
Lower Belgrave Street.

Miss K.V.B. Coni was one of the notable line of honorary treasurers of
the RCM (from 1947). In August 1964 the *Midwives' Chronicle* published a

short memoir she had written which touchingly describes the motives that impelled her to a career in midwifery education.

'From the age of seven I always hoped to be a trained nurse . . . I joined the Westminster Branch and had much help at the General Lying-in Hospital from Dr. Florence Willey and women medicals at the Royal Free Hospital. I consider the influence of the many famous women I met and heard speak, and the literature the movement produced, as some of the most formative and educational experiences of my life. On obtaining my hospital certificate in July 1917, I immediately arranged to take my midwifery training at the General Lying-in Hospital, York Road, Lambeth . . . It seemed to me stupid to be able to nurse medical and surgical cases and to be unable to help a woman in a natural emergency such as child-birth . . .

The General Lying-in Hospital was the pioneer in postgraduate teaching. This was inspired by Dr John Fairbairn and Miss Olive Haydon as head midwife. An annual week was held at the hospital which consisted of lectures and demonstrations, with attendance at ante-natal clinics (then in their infancy) also to the labour rooms and, if possible, the theatre. Milk kitchen demonstrations of prepared feeds were much prized.

Visits were paid to other maternity hospitals and departments, where unusual case histories and venereal diseases were included in talks and demonstrations. Approximately 100 midwives attended at their own volition and expense. The hospital charged 5s. to cover organising expenses and the occasional fee to a lecturer. The midwives provided their own accommodation and travelling expenses. It seems doubtful whether the free compulsory courses of today are as greatly appreciated. They continued to run for many years and were organised by Mrs. Mitchell as head midwife and by me as her successor . . .

In January 1924 I took up the post of matron of the Hull Municipal Maternity Hospital. The hospital was then in two semi-detached houses . . . The day after I arrived I was summoned to a meeting of the Local Authority's Health Committee. I was asked if I would take charge of the district service run by one midwife to whom two pupils from the hospital went for district experience. Only patients who could afford no fees attended.

The second important fact was then discovered – that the lease of the houses which formed the hospital was falling in at the end of February, and I was to move the hospital out to Cottingham and inhabit the first and only wing built for the future fever hospital which was standing empty.

I had two staff midwives, one of them was a pupil of mine appointed on the same day as myself, and one who was leaving in a month. Four pupils were approved for training, all of whom were half-way through their courses, and no vacancies had been filled. We were to increase from 14 beds to 30 beds. We had to improvise a labour ward and the staff were housed in the grounds in an army hutment.

Here we spent nearly five very happy years . . . In the meantime, I became a member of the Hull Association of Midwives (later the Hull Branch) and was elected President and Chairman in 1925 . . . In 1926 I was elected to the Council of the Royal College of Nursing. This kept me in touch with the Midwives Institute to whose Council I was also elected.'

Not surprisingly after surmounting these early difficulties Miss Coni went on to become a member of the CMB, a great teacher, and a reliable and accessible adviser to generations of officers and staff of the RCM.

The mid-sixties were a period of rapid and challenging change for the midwives. There was a time of uncertainty as the midwives had to readjust their methods of working to the new administrative structures. There was a real worry (as the 1964 Statement of Policy had indicated) that in the drive towards a tidy administrative pattern the personal and professional service of the midwife might become subsumed within general nursing. In particular, the absence of specific midwifery heads of departments in the hosptial plans meant that there was no career ladder available for midwives. In the event, midwives did climb the ladder of nursing promotion (Miss R.B. Worsley was appointed Chief Nursing Officer Grade 10 in the Portsmouth Group of Hospitals in 1969); but such successes were individual triumphs over the system as laid down.

Yet again the RCM had to fight for recognition for the midwives. Miss Foxton was succeeded as president in 1966 by Mrs Joan Goodman, and it was fitting that she should be the first president from the domiciliary side, having been non-medical Supervisor of Midwives for the London County Council, and later Borough Nursing Officer for midwives and district nursing in Lewisham. Her liveliness and enthusiasm were assets at a time when it was necessary for the midwives' case to be put clearly and forcefully. She was staunchly supported by Miss Audrey Wood, who as general secretary coped with the administrative burden of preparing and submitting evidence to committees of enquiry.

'When in doubt, form a committee' has always been a traditional British tactic, and it was employed over the reorganisation of the hospitals and health services. A Committee was formed by the Ministry of Health to examine the senior nursing staff structure in hospitals. This body (the Salmon Committee) reported in 1966 and, having given evidence to it, the RCM was able to welcome the Salmon recommendation that a midwifery division should be formed in each hospital district, and that each should be under the control of an experienced midwife. There was to be a new post of Chief Nursing Officer, whose main aim would be the coordination of policies affecting all types of nursing in hospitals; this officer would therefore have a voice in management, which was welcome. However, in laying down the qualifications for certain posts, Salmon excluded the midwife not also qualified as SRN from posts beyond Charge Nurse Grade 6; the RCM made representations to the Ministry. The main Salmon recommendations were accepted, and pilot schemes were set up in different parts of the country.

Pay and conditions of service for nurses and midwives were examined by the National Board for Prices and Incomes. Its report (No. 60), published in 1968, included the comment that 'It is widely felt that the nursing of mothers discharged after 48 hours could be undertaken by a home nurse/ maternity nurse under the supervision of a GP'. This extraordinary phrase, with its total misunderstanding of the continuity of care that had always been the essence of the midwife's function, caused profound resentment among midwives and was formally deplored by the AGM.

Greater sensitivity was demonstrated by the Health Services and Public Health Act 1968, which introduced greater flexibility into the administration of the health and social services.

The concept of a unified maternity service was at last accepted. Midwives might be employed by one authority, yet work in another, e.g. a domiciliary midwife employed by a local authority could continue her care of a woman when accompanying her to hospital and deliver her there. In other words, the function of the midwife was at last considered the most important criterion, rather than (as in the somewhat muddled administrative changes of the preceding decade) the place where she did her work. The barriers which had grown up between 'domiciliary' and 'hospital' midwives were breaking down. This was wholeheartedly welcomed by the RCM, and in 1968 the Statement of Policy was rewritten, omitting the words 'domiciliary' and 'hospital' in relation to midwives. It seemed that the principle of a unified service under an area health board was accepted.

Flexibility was also the RCM attitude to another controversial topic much debated at this time, in the wake of the Abortion Law Reform Bill introduced by David Steel MP. After long discussion, the RCM Council agreed to disagree on this contentious issue, and to leave the matter to the conscience of individual members. However, the RCM did formally support the 'conscience' clause proposed by (Sir) Bernard Braine MP.

As management responsibilities were being shouldered by more midwives, the RCM organised its first 'middle management' course at Mansfield Street in 1967–68. This was a one-year day release course for midwives and registered nurses with a minimum of five years' postgraduate experience. It was open to both male and female, and seventeen students followed that first course, of whom four were men.

Parallel with this, the RCM introduced a new subsidiary Council (added to those for supervisors, midwife teachers, and matrons) in 1968. This was the Council for Principal Midwife Teachers and Midwife Teachers in Charge, and was a further demonstration of the importance of management and training.

Three notable contributors to the midwives' cause died at the close of the 1960s. Miss Edith Elizabeth Greaves OBE died in October 1967 at the age of eighty-eight. She had been Matron of the City of London Maternity Hospi-

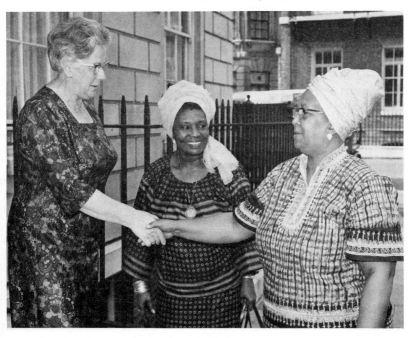

Miss Marjorie Bayes, executive secretary of the International Confederation of Midwives, welcomes visitors to 15 Mansfield Street

tal for thirty-four years (1912–1946) and nominee of the Ministry of Health on the CMB for twenty-seven years (1925–1952). She was a devoted member of the RCM, as chairman of the Matrons' Council and of the Education Committee, and played a considerable part in the foundation of the Midwife Teachers Training College. She was made an honorary vice-president of the RCM in 1952.

Sir Arnold Walker died in September 1968, aged seventy-one. Educated at Cambridge and the Middlesex Hospital, he became registrar to Sir Comyns Berkeley whom he was to succeed as chairman of the CMB. It was largely his intervention in 1941 which ensured that midwives were adequately represented on the National Advisory Council for the Recruitment and Training of Nurses and Midwives (afterwards the National Council of Nurses and Midwives). He was chairman of the Rushcliffe Midwives Salaries Committee, a vice-president of the RCM and a member of Council 1942 to 1968. In 1962 he generously presented to the RCM a fine Crown Derby tea set which had been a wedding present to his parents.

Mrs Florence Mitchell OBE, general secretary of the RCM from 1936–1952, died in February 1969. Following her retirement she had been elected a vice-president of the RCM in acknowledgement of her selfless and lifelong dedication; it was rightly said of her that 'when legislation affecting the wellbeing of mothers and babies or midwives was pending, she saw to it that the views of midwives were collated and expressed in the appropriate quarters. She worked for better standards of training and practice and better conditions of service. She recognised the need for postgraduate education and for special training for midwife teachers'.

The names of Sir Arnold Walker and Mrs Florence Mitchell are now commemorated in the name of the RCM library.

More formidable changes were signalled at the end of the sixties. Britain had failed to become a member of the European Economic Community (the Common Market) in the early years of the decade, but once again discussions were proceeding. Many professional bodies began to consider how the membership of a larger European community would affect them, and in particular how common standards of training and qualification might be achieved.

A European conference of midwives was held at the RCM in March 1969. It was opened by Miss Ellen Erup, chairman of the European Committee of the International Confederation of Midwives, and chaired by Sir John Peel, chairman of the Joint Study Group of the International Federation of Gynaecology and Obstetrics. The conference received reports from twenty-one countries; eighteen were represented by obstetricians, midwives and members of statutory bodies. The conference led later to the publication of the Copenhagen Report on the recruitment and training of midwives throughout Europe. This was one of the last events organised by Miss Marjorie Bayes, executive secretary of the International Confederation, while also deputy general secretary of RCM from which post she resigned that summer after twenty-seven years' service. Miss Bayes was awarded the Croix d'Officier par Merite et Dévouement Français for services to humanity, both for her work for the International Confederation and for her kindness to many generations of visiting students.

Miss Audrey Wood resigned as general secretary in 1970, after eighteen years. She had shouldered the burden of the immense changes during her years of office, but always with a deep respect for the democratic character of the RCM, and its reflection of opinion in the country as a whole.

It was said of her that she left behind her a body of women with trust in the College, and that was true. More perhaps than at any previous time the members felt that they had a voice at the centre. By a happy chance, Miss Wood's service was recognised at the Annual General Meeting at Belfast in 1970, where she was elected a Vice-President. Her earlier working life had been spent in Northern Ireland, where she was a vigorous secretary of the midwives' association in the province. She was awarded the OBE in the Birthday Honours of 1970. Miss Wood was succeeded as general secretary by Miss Brenda Mee who had been her assistant for the previous year. Belfast was also an appropriate site for that AGM for the newly-elected president of the RCM was Miss Rosemary Chesters Perkes, chairman of the

Northern Ireland Council, Matron of the Royal Maternity Hospital, Belfast from 1961.

There was to be no diminution of change. In 1969 the Redcliffe-Maud Commission on Local Government recommended a radical revision of local authorities, replacing the fragmented counties and boroughs with fewer but, it was hoped, more effective authorities. These changes were implemented by the Local Government Act of 1972 which came into effect on 1 April 1974. Once again the health services were subject to reorganisation.

Simultaneously but independently some of the health service trade unions began to threaten militant action in support of claims for better pay and conditions. Both the Royal College of Nursing and the RCM resolved in April 1970 that they would not strike in pursuit of wage claims, since this could only be a hazard to patients. Nevertheless the rates of pay and conditions of service of nurses and midwives were arousing concern, and in March 1970 the Secretary of State for the Social Services (the Rt Hon Richard Crossman) set up a Committee chaired by Professor Asa Briggs (then Vice-Chancellor of Sussex University) 'to review the role of the nurse and midwife in the hospital and the community and the education and training required for that role'.

The international reputation of British midwifery was demonstrated in 1971 by a request from Leipzig University, Warsaw for a print of the RCM film 'To Janet – a Son', made a decade earlier. Since then, the RCM had in fact produced another film, sponsored by Cow & Gate Ltd, on 'Midwifery in the UK'.

In the spring of 1971 the General Lying-in Hospital, York Road, closed its doors because of fewer maternity patients in the area, a reflection of the general decline of the inner cities. The hospital had been founded in 1765; its name was perpetuated in that of the 'Lambeth and General Lying-in Midwifery School' at St Thomas's Hospital.

In her presidential address to the Annual General Meeting of the RCM in July, Miss Perkes – who had been Matron of the 'G.L.I.' from 1954–61 – reflected on the many changes that had taken place since the passing of the last Midwives Act in 1936. Most strikingly, there was now a whole-time domiciliary service under the local health authorities. But in Britain nearly 100 per cent of all confinements took place within the hospital. Each domiciliary midwife's case-load averaged only twenty-seven babies annually, yet some of them were sometimes on call for sixty or eighty hours a week. Legislation had within three years integrated the domiciliary and hospital services.

'Together with the general practitioner, many domiciliary midwives undertake the care of the patient during pregnancy, take her into a GP unit for delivery, and providing everything appears normal, the same midwife takes the mother and baby home shortly afterwards. The continuity of care thus provided is not just by an individual midwife but by a team effort.'

This had been the type of procedure recommended by the Sub-Committee on Domiciliary Midwifery and Maternity Bed Needs (the Peel Committee) which had published its report shortly before.

Miss Perkes, who had received the OBE in the New Year Honours, was at that AGM wearing for the first time a new presidential badge – a reproduction of the coat of arms which had been attached to the chain of office bearing the names of past presidents (the old badge, attached to a blue ribbon, was subsequently worn on formal occasions by the chairman of Council).

The RCM, and the Midwives' Institute before it, was served by many devoted people who never aspired to high office, but without whose dedication much good work would not have been done. One such died in September 1971: Miss Winifred Burt, who was honorary secretary of the RCM Benevolent Fund for an astonishing forty-two years, from 1923 to 1965. Another was Mrs Renée Groves, who in 1973 retired from the editorship of the *Midwives' Chronicle* after twenty-two years.

At a time of great change, the Constitution of the RCM was an important stabilising factor. For the membership had a direct influence on the proceedings of the central Council, through their elected area representatives. Council consisted of sixty-one members; eleven National members, elected by ballot of the total membership, twenty-five area representatives, eight elected representatives from each of the advisory councils of the RCM, three representatives from Scotland, two from Northern Ireland, four vice-presidents, and the remainder co-opted members chosen for their particular skills and knowledge of the work of the RCM. The president, formally appointed at the Annual General Meeting, was nominated by Council and must have served on Council. Council elected its own chairman and vice-chairman, and the executive committee. Representatives were appointed to serve on such bodies as the CMB and the Nurses and Midwives Whitley Council.

It was not unusual for the presidency to go to a former chairman of Council, and it was so when in 1972 Miss Doris Hawkins succeeded Miss Perkes. She was Matron of the British Hospital for Mothers and Babies at Woolwich, founded by that former staunch member of the Midwives' Institute, Miss Alice Gregory. Miss Hawkins was forthright and business-like (she went to considerable trouble to ensure that all the proceedings of the RCM were correctly conducted). Very early in her period of office she was faced with another major change, when the Committee on Nursing chaired by Professor Asa Briggs reported in autumn 1972.

Briggs made seventy-five major recommendations for the nursing and midwifery services. The RCM had given detailed advice to the Committee and it was gratifying to see much of that advice reflected in the report. 'Particularly gratifying to midwives' (said the *Midwives' Chronicle*) 'will be the realisation that midwifery practice has paved the way for many of the

Committee's proposals, particularly their defined objectives with regard to the care of the patient, the code of practice as laid down by the CMB for England and Wales and the CMB for Scotland, the ability to adapt to changing technology, the statutory requirement for regular refresher courses, and in the great advance towards integration of the midwifery services between hospital and community which has already occurred'.

The main recommendation was that there should be a single central body, the Central Nursing and Midwifery Council, but with a statutory Standing Midwives Committee, a majority of whose members should be midwives. Midwives were to be represented 'in proper strength' both on the Central Council and on the three proposed national education boards. There were to be three distinct Boards for England, Scotland and Wales, all reporting to the Central Council. There would be area committees with boundaries coterminous with area health authorities or boards.

In responding to the Briggs proposals, which it did in Spring 1973, the RCM generally welcomed them. It was willing to accept the single Central Nursing and Midwives Council, but urged the distinct and separate identity of the midwifery profession. While agreeing to the setting up of area committees for nursing and midwifery education, the RCM accepted that the responsibility for such education should remain with the Department of Health and Social Security, the Scottish Home and Health Department and the World Health Organisation. But (and this point was reiterated many times in the negotiations that followed) 'Council wishes to ensure that the funds available to the Area Committees for educational purposes are entirely separate from those allocated to Area Health Boards for service needs'. The RCM was very familiar with the threat to education and training when the resources for it had to be found from general administrative budgets.

The RCM agreed with the two suggested ways of becoming a midwife: but 'if one year's practical experience is necessary after the one-year midwifery course to comply with EEC recommendations, then it would also be necessary after the 18 months' course'. The final decision for agreeing the content of courses should rest with the Standing Midwifery Committee. The RCM did disagree with proposals for 'crash' courses, though believed that there could be experiments with 'sandwich courses'.

Mature entrants to midwifery would be welcome, but in practice their contribution would be limited while their children were of school age. The RCM stressed the value of nursery nurses in midwifery. On staffing, there must be a balance between permanent and rotating night staff. Community nurses and midwives (as the 'domiciliary' staff were now styled) should work a defined number of hours each week, and 'on call' systems should be reviewed.

The Secretary of State (the Rt Hon Barbara Castle) accepted the main recommendations of Briggs in May 1974, and work began to implement them by legislation. The RCM was actively involved in the preparations for this.

In April 1973 the RCM could greatly rejoice when its honorary treasurer (the latest in a distinguished line holding that office, beginning with Dame Rosalind Paget herself) Miss Margaret Farrer D.N. (Lond) S.R.N. S.C.M. M.T.D., Chief Nursing Officer of the Thames Group Hospital Management Committee, was appointed first midwife chairman of the Central Midwives Board. At last, after seventy years, the statutory governing body of the profession had a midwife at its head.

It must have been a particular satisfaction to Miss Nora Deane, who survived to savour it. Miss Deane, probably the most remarkable of the post-war presidents, died later in April 1973 at the age of seventy. She had trained at the Prince of Wales Hospital, London, and then taken her midwifery training at the Rotunda, Dublin. In 1934 she became the youngest ever midwifery Matron, at Bristol. It was intended to close her hospital. Instead, she turned the Bristol Maternity Hospital into one of the leading training hospitals in the country. In 1963 Bristol University honoured her with an honorary degree. She was the first member of the nursing and midwifery professions to be president of the National Council of Women (1962–64).

She had been eager to encourage international cooperation, represented the RCM in Paris in 1953 when the first postwar International Congress was planned, and she presided over it in London in 1954. It was during her presidency that the Mansfield Street headquarters was planned, and partly through her drive and enthusiasm, built and opened. Appropriately, a memorial fund was opened, to enhance and improve the headquarters in her honour.

In 1972 the Scottish and Northern Ireland Councils of the RCM had changed their titles to become Boards; and in December 1973 a Welsh Board of the RCM was inaugurated at Cardiff. This was a particular satisfaction to one past president, Miss Mary Williams, whose pride in her Welsh origins was never hidden. The president and Council of RCM gave a dinner in Cardiff to make the inauguration, with the Minister of State for Wales (Mr David Gibson-Watt) as guest of honour.

As education was becoming still more important in the activities of the RCM, the staff was strengthened in January 1974 by the appointment as first director of education of Miss E. Anne Bent, and Miss Barbara Balch as Senior tutor in the education department with special responsibility for the course leading to the Advanced Diploma in Midwifery. Simultaneously Miss Virginia Rudwick became professional officer with responsibility for liaison with branches and the membership, and Mrs Katharine Szentpetery became family planning course organiser.

Industrial relations within the hospitals and health services, as elsewhere, became matters of sharp and sometimes bitter debate in these years. With the introduction of the Industrial Relations Act in 1971, the RCM registered on the special register for professional organisations. But inevitably, as the practice of midwifery was now so much concerned with the hospital environment, the sometimes militant dissension at various levels in the hospitals began to impinge upon the midwifery profession. To deal with this important matter a department of industrial relations was set up within the College, with Mrs A.M. Hardie as its first director.

This came to a head in 1974, when there were threats of strikes within the health service. The RCM held to its previous position. There would be no strike action by its members. There would be no withdrawal of labour in any form which could adversely affect patient care. There would be no mass resignations from the service.

Miss Hawkins, as president, faced the problem straightforwardly at the AGM that year.

'The main criticisms were that the College officers were old-fashioned, too ladylike and more concerned with speaking good English and wearing flowery hats than they were with getting good salaries and better conditions for midwives; that the College was running behind the larger organisations and taking what it could get for its members; and that the College was not heard or seen on radio, television or the press.'

The criticism about flowery hats was perhaps fair. The photographs of the officers of the RCM in the sixties do sometimes remind us more of hydrangeas than hygiene. But fashions change. The toques and voluminous black bombazine of the founders of the Midwives' Institute did not diminish their effectiveness or their concern, and nor did the flowery hats and twin-sets of a later generation.

The criticism that the RCM was 'running behind larger organisations' was grossly unfair to the general secretary, Miss Brenda Mee, who in fact was a member of the deputation from the staff side of the Whitley Council which on 20 May 1974 saw the Prime Minister (the Rt. Hon. Harold Wilson) with Mrs Barbara Castle (Secretary for Social Services), Mr Michael Foot (Secretary for Employment) and Mr Robert Hughes (Parliamentary Under-Secretary for Scotland). Two days later an independent review was announced, to be chaired by Lord Halsbury. Halsbury reported the following November, and proposed a simplification and improvement of the pay structure.

The integration of the midwifery services led to closer comparisons with nursing practice. The RCM therefore found itself fighting three battles: for the maintenance of professional recognition, and acknowledgement of the separate and distinct character of midwifery; the conferment of the status that the midwife deserved; and the demonstration of that status in salary scales. Some younger midwives, as some younger nurses, felt that the age required a more militant stance than the RCM as a professional organisation felt was necessary or desirable. But if the officers of the College did not take to the streets with banners, they were active in the committees and conferences where positive decisions were taken.

The integrated service made it more difficult for the College to devise a response to the Sex Discrimination Act of 1975. Some male nurses felt that they should have the right to take midwifery training. This was expressed,

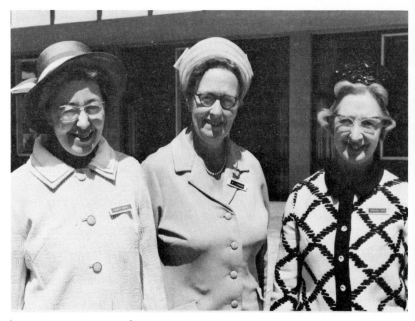

Left to right, Miss Audrey Wood, Miss Margaret Farrer and Miss Brenda Mee

for example, at a symposium organised by the South Worcestershire branch of the RCM in 1973, when one (male) speaker suggested that 'all nurses, both male and female, should as part of their general nursing training undertake a course of obstetric theoretical instruction and practical observation, the latter to include the witnessing of actual deliveries'.

When the Equal Opportunities legislation was effected, the RCM put forward the case that 'unless there is evidence that the majority of the public actually wishes to have male midwives, or that men would provide a more efficient or economic service, there are strong grounds for midwives to be listed under 'Exceptions' [to the law]. An independent attitude survey should be carried out to test public opinion on this matter'.

In a letter to the RCM in spring 1975 the Secretary of State (Mrs Barbara Castle) acknowledged that patients must have freedom of choice on the sex of the midwife; that male midwives would need chaperons; and that funds must be made available to meet the additional cost of employment of male midwives in the National Health Service. She continued: 'If Parliament accepts that the bar on male midwives should be removed, I can assure you that we will proceed very carefully in this field and in full consultation with the profession'.

A further consequence of integration was that the Hospital and Domiciliary Midwives Council had become an archaism; it was renamed the Branch Representative Council. Many of the problems facing the RCM in this period were common to other professional bodies. They came together in a Joint Committee of Professional Nursing and Midwifery Associations; and twelve bodies were represented at its inaugural meeting. The general secretary of the RCM, Miss Mee, became its honorary secretary.

In 1975 Miss M. McKivett retired from the service of the College after twenty-four years as tutor (in charge). That year also Miss Hawkins retired from the presidency after three extremely taxing years, and was succeeded by Mrs W. Agnes Andrews, who had been a supervisor of midwives in Birmingham for eighteen years and subsequently director of nursing services and then area nursing officer in Wolverhampton.

She was faced early by the problem of new trade union legislation. Under the new Trade Union and Labour Relations Act, the RCM would only be able to continue its function as a negotiating body for pay and conditions (as a member of the Whitley Council) if it registered as a trade union.

Following a resolution at the AGM in 1976, an Extraordinary General Meeting was called for 11 October. The response was so great that it had to be held at the Central Hall, Westminster: 890 members attended from all over the country. They were faced with a resolution to amend Clause 3 of the Articles of Association 'to apply to be placed on the list of trade unions maintained by the Certification Officer under the Trade Union and Labour Relations Act as amended, and thereafter to carry out the functions of a trade union as defined in that Act'. Three members voted against, with one abstention, and the resolution was therefore overwhelmingly carried.

There followed a necessary resolution 'to procure a subsidiary company to the College and the transfer of monies to it attributable to the charitable activities of the College'. The Royal College of Midwives Trust was then formed to carry on the educational and charitable functions of the RCM. That this move was approved by the membership at large was demonstrated by the result of a postal ballot which indicated that over 5,000 were in favour, and only 200 against.

The Queen Mother, as Patron, was informed of the proposed change and the reasons for it, and Her Majesty further agreed to continue to be Patron.

The College by 1977 represented 70 per cent of midwives in the country, and was thus in a strong position to make a submission to the Royal Commission on the National Health Service. The evidence put forward by the College was professional, detailed, and covered the full range of topics within the health service. As a preliminary, the College stated its endorsement of the definition of 'midwife' accepted by the Council of the International Confederation of Midwives five years earlier:

'A midwife is a person who, having been regularly admitted to a midwifery educational programme, duly recognised in the country in which it is located, has successfully completed the prescribed course of studies in midwifery and has acquired the requisite qualifications to be registered and/or legally licensed to practise midwifery. She must be able to give the necessary supervision, care and advice to women during pregnancy, labour and the postpartum period, to conduct deliveries on her own responsibility and to care for the newborn and the infant. This care includes preventive measures, the detection of abnormal conditions in mother and child, the procurement of medical assistance and the execution of emergency measures in the absence of medical help. She has an important task in health counselling and education, not only for patients but also within the family and the community. The work should involve antenatal education and preparation for parenthood and extends to certain areas of gynaecology, family planning and child care. She may practise in hospitals, clinics, health units, domiciliary conditions or in any other service.'

In its summary of evidence, the College laid down that the skills of the midwife should be fully utilised in the interests of the patients and for the best use of available resources; clarification of the role of each member of the maternity services team was essential.

The maternity liaison committees were not successful before the NHS reorganisation, partly because of lack of cooperation by medical staff. The health care planning teams did not appear to be making any better progress, supposedly for similar reasons. The College argued that schemes to link maternity grants and benefits (which could amount to £250 for the first baby) to professional care should be considered: the Swedish scheme offered a precedent. The mother wished to be able to choose where she went for prenatal and intranatal care, and when in the postnatal period she might be transferred home: in some units arbitrary uniform decisions on the latter were made by medical staff. Financial manpower and other resources should be made through divisional midwifery budgets to enable health education to be available throughout the maternity services.

On forward planning, the College called for great flexibility. Noting that new technologies were introducing new diagnostic techniques and active management of labour, the College emphasised that these did not decrease midwifery staffing levels, or the need for clinical skills. Midwives needed to acquire additional knowledge and expertise, and the patient required additional emotional support and information.

On service to patients, the College upheld its traditional belief that the community and hospital midwifery service should remain in one division, with a practising midwife at its head. The Royal Commission was asked to consider bringing the family practitioner within the remit of community health councils; all general practitioner obstetricians and their locums should be qualified and experienced in obstetrics. The interface between the NHS and the personal social services was vital. 'With the current emphasis on a shift to increased care in the community the need for effective joint planning is essential'; the integration of health and social services under a single administration, as in Northern Ireland, could be considered.

On the management of the NHS, the College submitted that the principle of consensus team management should remain, since it was the experience of members of the College that it could function effectively. There might be too many tiers of management between those responsible for resource allocation and those delivering the service, and there should be clarification of roles. In the nurse membership of health authorities and boards, there should be a clear distinction between the nurse worker member and the nurse who is contributing professional expertise, and both should be represented.

Finally on the resources of the NHS, the College submitted that before decisions concerning manpower levels were made particular attention should be given to the disparity in existing staffing levels in a comparable unit, and unacceptable working levels resulting from using standard calculations without reference to the size and design of wards and departments. The College Annual General Meeting had resolved in 1976 that finance for midwifery education should be separate from service funds. The College considered that there was a great need for examination of the balance of expenditure between direct delivery of care and administrative support, community based care *vis-à-vis* hospital based care, and preventive services and acute services. The cost of new equipment also concerned the College, since this was said to reduce costs, but in fact often introduced new costs in terms of maintenance, servicing and associated staffing levels. Lastly, the College deprecated the lack of provision by the NHS of an occupational health service for its employees; such services in industry had demonstrated their cost-effectiveness.

When the Royal Commission reported (in July 1979) it had taken account of much of the RCM evidence; indeed, its report contained the crucial statement that 'midwifery has long been recognised as a separate profession, although the majority of midwives are also trained nurses . . . The role of the midwife may serve as a model of the extended role and clinical responsibility which nurses could carry'.

Among the recommendations were an occupational health service for NHS employees; research into the effect of the use of unqualified nursing staff on patient care; the establishment of budgets for post-basic nursing education; improved career structures for clinical nurses and midwives; the development of the clinical role of the nursing officer; and peer review of standards of care for the health professions by the professional bodies including the Royal Colleges.

Many of these recommendations – budgets for education, improved career structures, and the advice of the Royal Colleges in assessing standards of care – had been RCM policy for many years.

The Briggs Committee on nursing midwifery practice and education had reported in 1972, and been accepted by the Government. But no legislation followed. Then, after six years, it seemed possible that legislation would appear. As chairman of the CMB, Miss Farrer expressed the Board's concern at the suggestion throughout the report that the professions of nursing and midwifery should be fused. She pointed out the considerable changes that had taken place in six years: devolution, the reorganisation of the NHS, EEC directives to coordinate practice and training throughout the Community, and changes in national employment legislation.

An Extraordinary meeting of the RCM Council was held on 20 February 1978 to review the proposed legislation. At its second reading in the House of Commons on 13 November, it seemed likely to go through with less security for midwives than at any time in the past eighty years. Then, in the committee stage, following representations from the RCM, the Minister of State (Health), Mr Roland Moyle, put forward a new clause relating to the statutory Midwives Committee of the Nurses, Midwives and Health Visitors' Council:

'1) Of the members of the Council's Midwifery Committee the majority shall be practising midwives.
2) The Council shall consult the Committee on all matters relating to midwifery.
3) The Council shall assign to the Committee all matters relating to midwifery.
4) The Secretary of State shall not approve rules relating to midwifery practice unless satisfied that they are framed in accordance with recommendations of the Council's Midwifery Committee.
5) Any matter which is assigned to the Midwifery Committee otherwise than under subsection (3) shall be finally dealt with by the Committee on behalf of the Council.'

The Bill received its third reading on 7 February 1979 and was one of a number of pieces of legislation which received the Royal Assent shortly before the proroguing of Parliament on 4 April. Once again the status and conditions of service of the midwives had been saved by the hard and persistent efforts of its leaders. Not least among them on this occasion was Miss Margaret Farrer, a notable speaker, who in April 1979 retired as chairman of the CMB after six years (and twenty-seven years as a member of the Board). She was succeeded as chairman by Miss N.M. Hickey.

Simultaneously with all this activity, the apparently indefatigable Miss Mee was with her customary good humour coping with a great amount of work while with Miss Annie Grant, education officer of the CMB Scotland, representing the RCM in negotiations over the status of the midwife, her training and reciprocity within the European Economic Community: the 'EEC directives'. She also prepared the RCM's submission, in August 1979, to the Standing Committee on Nurses and Midwives Pay Comparability (the Clegg Commission).

The AGM was held in Glasgow in July 1979, and members were welcomed by Miss M.M. Grieve M.B.E., chairman of the Scottish board. Members had deeply considered the question of affiliation to the Trade

Union Congress; but not least because many members were disquieted by the suggestion that, following affiliation, there might be pressure to merge with other unions, it was decided that 'no further action be taken at this time but that Council continues to monitor the situation and explore further alternatives'.

Following the AGM, Miss Mee and her secretary and friend Miss Hazel Allen went for a camping holiday in north Wales. They were walking near the top of Snowdon when they appear to have slipped and fallen to their deaths. This tragedy was a profound blow to the RCM and its members. Miss Brenda Mee, who was 53, had been awarded the OBE in 1977. She had formerly been superintendent midwife at Kingston Hospital, and previously at Rochford, before joining the RCM staff as assistant secretary in 1968, and general secretary from 1971. During those nine years she had dealt with a multitude of problems and challenges with dedication and thoroughness but she was also remembered for her infectious laugh, and her ability to keep a sense of proportion in the most difficult times.

The contribution she made to the RCM was defined by the president, Mrs Andrews, at her memorial service in the parish church of the College, All Souls, Langham Place.

'The 1970s have been times of great change in society and in the National Health Service through which Brenda, with her vision, has steered the College, always keeping foremost the interest of midwives and midwifery . . . At the same time she was able to identify issues which were important for other professions and the areas where cooperation was essential for the good of the service, and therefore of the public.

She had the ability to detect trends and to grasp quickly and with clarity new and important issues. A striking example of these were developments in the industrial and educational fields . . . Her careful watchfulness and advice culminated in the almost unanimous decision by members of the College in 1976 to apply for certification as a trade union. Another result of her foresight was the establishment of the Labour Relations Department at the College. Her interest in developments in general education and in the nursing and health visiting fields, and the need which she recognised for progress in midwifery education, led among other things to the reorganisation of the education department in the College and her enthusiasm as a founder member of the Joint Board of Clinical Nursing Studies.

She has been one of the two RCM representatives of the EEC Midwives Liaison Committee since 1971, when the College was invited to become a member of this Committee. She was elected secretary to the Committee in 1974, a post which she held until her death. The progress which has been made in the difficult negotiations of the EEC Midwives Directives, and the understanding of the problems of the midwives of the EEC countries, is in no small measure due to her indefatigable work.'

The nine years during which Brenda Mee was general secretary of the RCM were certainly the most difficult in the history of the College. New

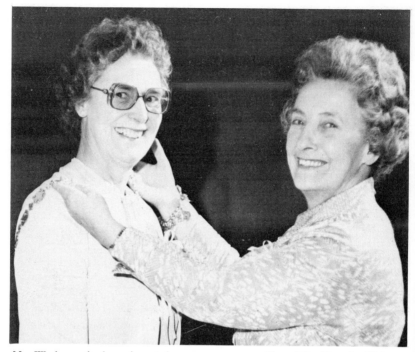

Mrs W. Agnes Andrews invests her successor as president, Miss Dorothy Webster, with the chain of office, 16 July 1980

challenges – in industrial relations, in administrative changes, in the changed relationship of Britain with Europe – posed problems that were unprecedented. Each was faced and overcome.

The months following Brenda Mee's death were naturally overshadowed by this tragedy. She had been, essentially, a practical and most active midwife, who had brought her sense of realism to the service of this institution.

Eventually, to succeed her the Council chose a young midwife who in her posts as tutor in the education department and as professional officer of the RCM had gained experience in the working of headquarters. Miss Ruth Ashton took up the office of general secretary in 1980.

In succession to Mrs Andrews, Miss Dorothy Webster became president in 1980, as the preparations to celebrate the centenary began. It was by a happy coincidence that the midwives of Britain, in this celebratory year, would play host to the midwives of the world; for the nineteenth International Congress of the International Confederation of Midwives was planned to be held in Brighton in September 1981.

This outward-looking spirit would surely have delighted the founders, those remarkable women who a century ago set up the 'Midwives' Institute' to encourage the training of midwives so as to lead to a better standard of

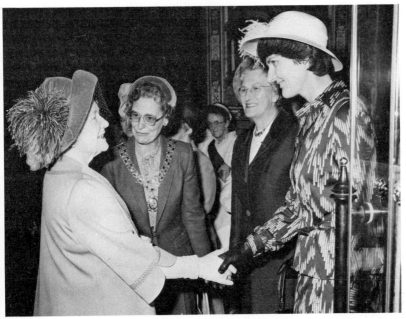

Her Majesty the Queen attends the Royal College of Midwives centenary service at Westminster Abbey, April 1981

care for mothers and babies. Some of the activities of the RCM today they would probably find surprising. That it should be a trade union, and conduct negotiations over pay and conditions, is probably more than they could imagine. But that the RCM should be so profoundly concerned with education and training is something they would certainly applaud; and that it should be done by the active cooperation of many thousands of midwives from all parts of the country, England, Scotland, Wales and Northern Ireland, is the ideal at which they aimed.

It was their belief that every mother should have the right to the highest standards of care during the most critical period in her and her baby's life. They campaigned strongly and persistently to that end, as their successors have had to do, and continue to do, to this day. They would be proud of the Royal College of Midwives. They would note that it has maintained its standards, and improved them, by constant care and constant vigilance.

VITA DONUM DEI

OFFICERS
OF THE ROYAL COLLEGE OF MIDWIVES
(formerly the Midwives' Institute)

PRESIDENTS

1881–1894 Zepherina Smith	1958–1960 Mary Williams OBE
1894–1911 Jane Wilson	1960–1963 Jean P. Ferlie OBE
1911–1919 Amy Hughes	1963–1966 Frances R. Foxton
1919–1926 Anne Campbell Gibson	1966–1970 Joan M. Goodman
1926–1928 Lucy Ramsden	1970–1972 Rosemary C. Perkes OBE
1928–1949 Edith M. Pye, Chev.d'Hon.	1972–1975 Doris M. Hawkins OBE
1949–1952 Mabel Liddiard CBE	1975–1980 W. Agnes Andrews CBE
1952–1958 Nora Deane CBE	1980 Dorothy Webster

CHAIRMEN OF COUNCIL*

1944–1947 Miss E. Pye	1965–1966 Mrs J. Goodman
1947–1948 Mrs A. Baker	1966–1969 Miss Z.M. Goodall
1948–1951 Miss N.B. Deane MBE	1969–1972 Miss D.M. Hawkins OBE
1951–1954 Miss E.F. Gore	1972–1975 Mrs W.A. Andrews OBE
1954–1957 Miss M. Williams	1975–1978 Miss A.S. Grant OBE
1957–1960 Miss F.R. Foxton	1978–1980 Miss D.M. Webster
1960–1962 Miss E.K. Bally	1980–1981 Miss J. Beak
1962–1965 Miss M. Farrer	

* It would appear that before 1944, the president took the chair at Council meetings.

GENERAL SECRETARIES

1936 Mrs F.R. Mitchell OBE SCM
1952 Miss A. Wood OBE BA SRN SCM MTD
1970 Miss B. Mee OBE SRN SCM MTD
1980 Miss R. Ashton SRN SCM MTD

Index